Essential Oils Box Set For Specific Individuals

For Beginners, Kids And Babies, Family Health And Pets (4 books in 1)

CORAL MILLER

Copyright © 2015 Coral Miller

All rights reserved. No part of this publication may be reproduced, distributed, or transmitted in any form or by any means, including photocopying, recording, or other electronic or mechanical methods, without the prior written permission of the publisher, except in the case of brief quotations embodied in critical reviews and certain other noncommercial uses permitted by copyright law.

ISBN-13:978-1512262759

ISBN-10:1512262757

Disclaimer

The information in this book is solely for informational purposes, not as a medical instruction to replace the advice of your physician or as a replacement for any treatment prescribed by your physician. The author and publisher do not take responsibility for any possible consequences from any treatment, procedure, exercise, dietary modification, action or application of medication which results from reading or following the information contained in this book.

If you are ill or suspect that you have a medical problem, we strongly encourage you to consult your medical, health, or other competent professional before adopting any of the suggestions in this book or drawing inferences from it.

This book and the author's opinions are solely for informational and educational purposes. The author specifically disclaims all responsibility for any liability, loss, or risk, personal or otherwise which is incurred as a consequence, directly or indirectly, of the use and application of any of the contents of this book.

DEDICATION

To my husband, Kirk, Thank you for standing by me.

TABLE OF CONTENTS

INTRODUCTION TO THE BOX SET 17
BOOK 1 19
CHAPTER 1 20
    All About Essential Oils 20
    Application And Dosage 25
    Storage And Care 26
    Using Essential Oil Correctly 27
CHAPTER 2 32
    Top Essential Oils For Every Beginner 32
    Lavender 32
    Lemon 33
    Peppermint 35
    Sandalwood 37
    Tea Tree 38
CHAPTER 3 40
    Recipes For Body & Skin Care 40
CHAPTER 4 53
    Recipes For Hair Care 53
CHAPTER 5 58
    Recipes For Emotional Well Being 58
CHAPTER 6 63
    Recipes For Household 63

CHAPTER 7 71
Other Essential Oil Recipes 71
Beauty, Aromatherapy, Pets And More 71

BOOK 2 81

INTRODUCTION 82
Essential Oils, Aromatherapy And Your Kid..82
Benefits Of Essential Oils For Kids And Babies....................................83
Using Essential Oils Safely 84
Using Essential Oils For Children...85
Essential Oils That Are Good For Children..87

REMEDIES FOR COMMON AILMENTS 90
General Guidelines For Dilution..90
Fever..90
Sunburn...90
Colds and Runny Nose...91
Flu..91
Diaper Rash..91
Common Cold Blend 92
Bruises 93
Minor Burns 93
Colic Blend..93
Cradle Cap 94
Crying 94
Chicken Pox..95
Cuts And Scrapes...95
Coughs..96

 Diarrhea 96

 Hiccoughs 96

 Jaundice 97

 Earache 97

 Insect Bites 98

 Constipation 98

 Teething 98

 Tummy Ache 99

 Rashes 99

 Sleeping 100

MASSAGE OILS AND LOTIONS 101

 Homemade Baby Oil 101

 Baby Balm 101

 Diaper Cream 102

 Soft Baby Oil 103

 Homemade Lotion for Babies 104

 Nourishing Baby Lotion 105

 Rich Baby Oil 106

 Homemade Diaper Balm 107

 Baby Smooth Balm 108

HYGIENE AND BATH 109

 Homemade Shampoo & Body Wash 109

 Lavender Baby Shampoo 109

 Baby Powder 110

 Chamomile Baby Shampoo 110

 Teething Gel 111

Milk Bath 111
Homemade Baby Powder 112
Homemade Baby Wipes 112
Baby Healing Wipes 113
Baby Bubble Bath 114
SUNSCREEN LOTIONS 115
Homemade Sunscreen 115
Natural Homemade Sunscreen 116
INSECT REPELLENTS FOR CHILDREN 117
Homemade Insect Repellent 117
Water Based Bug Spray 118
Oil Based Bug Spray 119
Patchouli Bug Spray 119
Wonder Bug Spray 120
Citronella Spray 120
Soothing Insect Spray 121
Itchy Relief Repellent 122
HOUSE CLEANING 123
Homemade Laundry Soap 123
Homemade Liquid Laundry Soap 124
Perfect Stain Remover 125
Boom Liquid Dishwasher 125
Homemade Toy Cleaner 126
Homemade Surface Cleaner 126
Safe Surface Cleaner 127
Citrus Surface Cleaner 127

BOOK 3 128
INTRODUCTION 129
    Why Essential Oils Are So Powerful 130
    Quality Of Essential Oils 131
    How To Use Essential Oils 132
    Top Essential Oils For Healing 134
COLDS & COUGHS 138
    Cough Mixture 138
    Vapor Rub 138
    Power Chest Rub 139
    Colds 140
    Colds & Flu Home Spray 140
    Anti-Flu Bath 141
    Anti- Flu Massage 141
    Cold Sores Quick Fix 141
    Cold Sores Blend 142
    Kid's Cold Cure 142
    Nasal Inhaler 143
    Ease Sinus Congestion 143
    Night-Time Colds & Flu Combater 143
SKIN INJURIES & BOO-BOOS 145
    Blisters 145
    Grazes 145
    Emergency Burn Wash/Compress 146
    Bruise 146
    Minor Burns 146

Insect Bites 147

Insect Repellent Spray 147

Antiseptic Cream 147

Wounds 148

Bleeding 149

Cuts Spray 149

Boils 150

Anti- Abscess Compress 150

HEADACHES 151

Fast Fix Remedy 151

Anti- Headache Blend 151

Tension/ Nervous Headache Mix 152

Headache Balm 152

STOMACH RELIEF 153

Diarrhea 153

Hiccups 153

Stomach Massage 154

Nausea Instant Remedy 154

Motion Sickness 155

Heartburn 155

Bladder Infection Oil 155

Bladder Infection Sitz Bath 156

PAINS 157

For Rheumatism & Arthritis 157

Massage Oil For Abdominal Pain 157

Massage Oil Remedy 158

Cramp 158

Bedsores 158

Bedsore Massage Oil 159

ORAL HEALTH 160

Mouth Ulcers 160

3. Power Mouthwash 160

Gum Strengthener 161

Bad Breath 161

Chapped Lips 162

Toothache 162

Massage Oil For Toothache 163

SKIN CARE REMEDIES 164

For Stretch Marks 164

Sunburn Soother 164

Gentle Wart Removal 164

Blemish Blocker 165

Easy Facial Toner 165

Facial Toner 166

Intensive Blemish Treatment 166

FEVER 167

Fever Massage Blend 167

EYE CARE 168

Sty 168

Conjunctivitis Compress 168

EAR, NOSE & THROAT 169

Catarrh 169

- Hay Fever 169
- Catarrh Rub 170
- Pain Relief For Earache 170
- Sinusitis Steam Inhalation 171
- Massage Oil For Sinusitis 171
- Nosebleed 172

BODY ACHES & PAINS 173
- Muscle Pain 173
- Nerve Pain Oil 173
- Back Pain Massage 174
- Aromatherapy Bath 174

LOWER BLOOD PRESSURE 174

EMOTIONAL HEALTH 175
- Insomnia Blend 175
- Insomnia Remedy 175
- Jetlag 176
- Release Sexual Energy 176
- Comfort the Bereaved 177
- Fatigue Fader 177
- Concentration Spray 178

BOOK 4 179

INTRODUCTION 180
- Essential Oils And Your Pet 180
- Diluting Essential Oils For Dogs 182
- Essential Oils Benefits for Fido 183
- Safe Essential Oils For Dogs 184

Essential Oil Precautions With Dogs 186
   How To Apply Essential Oils To Dogs 187
ESSENTIAL OIL DOG BATH RECIPES 188
   Calming Shampoo 188
   Puppy Shampoo 188
   Tick Repelling Shampoo 189
   Flea/ Insect Repelling Shampoo 189
   Spicy Deodorant Shampoo 190
   Tender Floral 190
   Citrus Refreshing Shampoo 191
   Herbal Fresh Shampoo 191
ESSENTIAL OILS FOR DOGS' EARS 193
   Lavender Wax Cleanser 193
   Doggie Ear Mites 194
   Dog Ear Infection 194
   Power Ear Infection Blend 195
SKIN AND COAT ISSUES 196
   Dog Burns 196
   Deodorizing Spray 196
   Dog Abscess 197
   Calming Mist Spray 197
   Rich Fragrant Shampoo 198
   Wound Blend 199
   Dog Growths 199
   Doggie Anti-Itch Blend 199
   Insect Bite Blend 200

Itchy Skin Remedy 201

Bad Odor Remedy 201

Power Odor Spray 202

FLEAS AND TICKS 203

Natural Tick Spritzer 203

Oregano Tick Removal 203

Flea Control 204

Tick Repellent 204

Flea and Deodorizing Collar 205

Anti Fleas Shampoo 205

Mosquito Repellent 206

ESSENTIAL OILS FOR EMOTIONS 207

For Calming Dogs 207

For Girl Crazy Dogs 207

For Hyperactive Dogs 207

Anxiety Oil Blend 208

For Nervous Exhaustion 209

Calming Powder Blend 209

ESSENTIAL OIL FOR BONE ISSUES 210

Joint Pain Relief Blend 210

Doggie Aging Ointment 210

Arthritis Relief 211

ESSENTIAL OILS FOR MICELLANEOUS ISSUES 212

Immune Support for Allergens 212

Sunburned Nosed Dog 212

Sinus Infections 212

Carsick Dogs/ Colic 213
For Brain Health Support.. 213
Respiratory Support 214
Dog With A High Fever... 214
Motion Sickness 214

INTRODUCTION TO THE BOX SET

Everyone needs to know how to use essential oils. They are useful for a wide range of applications, providing lots of healing, cleansing and soothing benefits when used correctly. To me, I consider them indispensable. In my research, however, I discovered that they are limited information on specific usage. So I decided to focus on those areas through the release of my four books so a whole lot of people can benefit.

I am glad that the release of my essential oils books in four parts has been a blessing to a large audience. However, I sincerely believe that a considerable number can still be reached through the release of this box set and at a much lower cost.

Here In This Box Set Are My Four Essential Oil Books:

Book 1: Essential Oils For Beginners: Easy Step By Step Guide With Recipes For Skin Care, Hair care, Emotional Wellbeing, Household Use And More

Book 2: Essential Oils For Kids And Babies: A Simple Guide To Aromatherapy And Using Essential Oils For Children

Book 3: Essential Oils For Family Health: Simple Aromatherapy Recipes For Common Ailments

Book 4: Essential Oils For Your Pet: 47 Safe, Natural And Easy Home Remedies For Fido (Aromatherapy for Dogs)

The table of contents has not been changed but simply combined to make it much easier for you to get what you need. However, each book in this box set retains its introductory page where necessary so you could enjoy a wholesome package.

This box set, 'essential oil for specific individuals', ends your search.

For Beginners, get the basic knowledge, tips, recipes and remedies that you need to get you started.

For Kids And Babies, parents can now learn how to use essential oils to treat diaper rash and various minor baby ailments and also use these oils in beauty products such as cleansers, powders, oils and baby wipes to ensure a happy and healthy child.

For Family Health, learn how to treat common ailment at home and keep your family healthy all year long.

For Pets, learn how your dog can enjoy the healing and comforting remedies of essential oil. Have a healthy, happy Fido that you can always hang around with.

You will be so glad you purchased this book!

Coral Miller

BOOK 1

Essential Oils For Beginners

Easy Step By Step Guide With Recipes For Skin Care, Hair care, Emotional Wellbeing, Household Use And More

Coral Miller

CHAPTER 1

All About Essential Oils

Essential oils are natural, highly concentrated aromatic liquids that are extracted from the flowers, leaves, roots, fruits, shrubs, seeds, bushes of various plants. They are powerfully and beautifully fragrant, providing plants with their distinct aroma and enhancing their immune system. They provide plants with protection against harmful insects, disease and harsh environmental conditions. They are natural alternatives for overall health care and general well being.

Essential oils have been in use from ancient times; as far back as 4500 BC. The early people had stumbled into certain plants that could cure their common ailments. They went further to concentrate these plant essences into essential oils which they used in treating illnesses, in religious rituals and as perfumery.

They passed this discovery to their descendants and over the years, there have been lots of improvement in its usage. Today, research has proven that essential oils, besides being safer and more affordable, work just as well and in some cases even better than commercial products. Essential oils are now used for numerous emotional and physical wellness applications.

Essentials oils are not really oils in the real sense of the word as they do not feel oily. They are not like our cooking oils either. The reason they are called "oils" is the high number of oil-soluble chemicals present in the plant (about 100-200 chemicals in one essential oil). They are highly concentrated, even much more potent than dried herbs. For instance, 1 drop of peppermint oil equals 26 cups of peppermint tea in potency and 1 drop of lemon oil equals 16 lemon rinds as well!

Since essential oils are extracted straight from parts of plants or trees, they possess a complex nature that is hard to replicate outside of nature. Actually, some essential oils contain substances that do not occur naturally anywhere else. Furthermore, they are not the same as fragrance oils. Fragrance oils are artificially created perfumes which have been infused with synthetic scents for aesthetic effect. Essential oils, on the other hand, actually provide the natural therapeutic benefits of their original plants.

When purchasing essential oils, make sure they are pure and of high quality. Do not buy fragrance oils or diluted essentials oils. The therapeutic properties are in the actual substances and not just the fragrance. Cheap copies bring cheap results, causing problems like skin irritation or even worsening an already existing ailment. There is no regulating body for essential oils so make sure you buy from reputable sources to get your money's worth. To test if your oils are pure, put 3-4 drops on a blotting paper. Once evaporated, pure essential oils will not leave any residue but petroleum solvents and adulterated essential oils will.

Like any other substances, safety precautions must be taken when using essential oils. When using any essential oil for the first time, carry out a skin patch test. This test will also help you to know if you have a sensitive skin or you have an allergy to the oil.

To do a skin patch test, dilute your essential oil in carrier oil. Place 1-2 drops on the inner side of your upper arm, cover with a bandage and keep it dry for 24 hours. If the skin turns red or feels hot, then it is unsafe for your use. Apply vegetable oil to the area to dilute the essential oil. You can also wash it immediately with water and mild soap but this is less effective. Do not overlook this procedure as it is essential. Additionally, do not take anybody's word for it because two people may react differently to essential oil applied on them. Also remember that if you are allergic to any plant, you are likely to be allergic to its essential oil.

Like regular tanning oils, essential oils if not carefully used can cause sunburn or even very deep burns. If it gets into your eyes, dampen a cotton cloth with sesame or olive oil and apply it to your eyelids. Be informed that some essential oils can irritate the eyes so must be used with care. Again, a few can be poisonous e.g. tea tree oil. Avoid this poisonous essential oil for mouthwash.

The safest way to treat essential oil is to consider them as medicines. This way, you will be able to lessen the level of harm that may occur, if handled wrongly.

Other Safety Guidelines Include:

• Do not use undiluted essential oils on your skin. With the exception of lavender and tea tree oils (Melaleuca), on no account should you use any essential oil in its pure form.

• Do not use essential oil without the counsel of your physician if you are pregnant. Additionally, individuals with health conditions like epilepsy and asthma must seek a doctor's approval.

• Do not exceed the recommended dosage for essential oils. Remember it is very strong and the smallest amount can still get the job done.

• Essential oils are flammable so protect from fire hazards.

• Not all essential oils can be used in aromatherapy. Pennyroyal, Wormood, Camphor, Onion, Sassafras, Horseradish, Bitter Almond and Rue are some of these essential oils.

• Keep all essential oils should out of children's reach. Do not be carried away with the fragrances emitting from these oils to forget that they can be hazardous in young children's hands.

• Do not use essential oils on damaged or chemically- burned skin.

• Wash hands thoroughly after application so you do not leave essential oil residue on your fingers. This may damage contact lenses and cause eye discomfort.

• Do not put essential oils directly into the ears, nose and avoid getting it in to your eyes.

• To prevent inflammation or itchy skin, wear disposable latex gloves when working with them.

• Always work in an area with good ventilation.

Essential oils are the major ingredients in aromatherapy treatments. There are more than 100 different types in the market. Amazingly, each of these oils contains its own special scent and properties that are applicable to many different conditions. Here are some popular essential oils and their uses:

• **Eucalyptus**: invigorating and purifying, it is often used in topical preparations but do not apply to children's face.

• **Ginger**: helps to stimulate the appetite and relieves headaches.

• **Lavender**: promotes a relaxed and calm feeling.

• **Lemon**: joyful oil that also refreshes but should be diluted well if applying to the skin.

• **Peppermint**: filled with powerfully minty aroma, peppermint oil is refreshing and cooling.

• **Rosemary**: This clarifying fragrance is generally used in shampoos, household sprays and soaps.

• **Sage**: has a warming camphor scent and you need just one drop to experience it.

• **Tea Tree**: helps to fight against bacteria, viruses and fungi and stimulate the body's immune system.

• **Ylang Ylang**: originally cultivated in the Philippines, the ylang ylang plant soon became widespread due to its distinctive scent and look. This essential oil helps to relax the mind and body.

• **Clove** a versatile oil, it provides relief from aches and pains such as headache, tooth and gum pain, earache and stomach ache. It is also useful for skin ailments such as bug bites and cuts.

Kid- friendly essential oils include lavender, lemon, grapefruit, pine, tea tree, spruce and peppermint for kids above 6 years of age.

Carrier Oils

Carrier oils are cold-pressed vegetable oils from plant's fatty parts. They help to dilute the highly concentrated essential oils before they are applied onto the skin as undiluted essential oils can cause burning and irritation. Unlike essentials oils, they do not evaporate and contain little or no aroma. However, they have a shorter life span.

They can be used for bath oils, massages, creams, lip balms and lotions. Carrier oils must always be used with babies, small children and individuals with sensitive skin. They should also be unadulterated and as natural as possible.

There are various carrier oils with different properties and features. Your preferred choice will depend on your desired therapeutic benefit. Below are some carrier oils and their benefits.

Types of Carrier Oils

Coconut Oil (Fractionated) – one of the best natural moisturizer, this oil is great for dry environments.

Jojoba Oil- Jojoba – absorbs easily into the skin.

Sweet almond oil– helps the skin to maintain its elasticity, promotes better circulation and is a natural UV blocker.

Hemp seed oil – great moisturizer oil that prevents brittle hair.

Hazelnut oil –helps to prevent eczema and acne.

Apricot kernel oil– one of the best for creating skin-healing oil blends, it helps to hydrate and nourish the skin and encourage skin cells' regeneration.

Others include grapeseed oil, olive oil, avocado oil, cranberry seed oil, sunflower seed oil, macadamia nut oil, sesame oil and evening primrose oil.

Application And Dosage

Use essential oils sparingly and do not exceed the recommended dosage as they are very potent. As little as 1 to 2 drops will go a long way towards offering the therapeutic benefits that is required.

The most effective and safest area of the body for applying essential oils is the bottom of the feet. This is very helpful for young children or people with frail health. The sole of our feet are thick and are unlikely to cause skin irritations. Thus, the feet are really great place to apply "hotter" oils and anti-infectious blends.

Also, there are lots of nerve endings on the soles of the feet which help to carry the oils quickly into the bloodstream. For example, if you rub a clove of garlic clove on the bottom of your foot, your breath will smell of garlic within 15 minutes!

To treat a particular area like a rash, burn, wound or sore muscle, apply the oils on the problem spot directly. Other safe areas for applying oils are the inside elbows and knees, the nape of the neck and base of the throat.

Another good area for applying essential oils is the scalp because the size of the hair follicle is much bigger than the skin pores. Essential oils penetrate the scalp easily when it is applied on it, stimulating it.

Essential oils can last between 12 - 24 hours in the body. However, certain factors such as the body area where the oils were applied, the application method (topical or inhalation), viscosity and skin type can diminish or extend the therapeutic duration.

Storage And Care

Essential Oils evaporate quickly which is why they are termed "volatile". To avoid evaporation, they must be kept sealed airtight in dark colored bottles (away from ultra violet light) and away from heat. Store them in a cool, dry and dark place. By sealing airtight, the essential oils' volatile components are contained within the bottle, oxidation is prevented and the traditional healing properties of the oils are retained.

While essential oils do not come with an expiration date, optimum shelf life is about two years. Most lose some of their potency after this but citrus essential oils such as lime and orange usually degrade quickly (six month shelf life). A few essential oils like Jasmine, Cypress, Rose and Patchouli actually become more potent as they age. Always write the date of purchase on the essential oil bottle.

Refrigerating essential oils isn't really necessary. Except for rose, it may even be detrimental because some essential oils are as solid as can be at low temperatures.

Using Essential Oil Correctly

There are 3 basic ways to use essential oils: topical application, inhalation, and internal consumption. Depending on the user's experience and desired benefit, essential oils can be used as single oil or in blends.

1. **Topical Application**

The skin absorbs essentials oil easily. Therefore, it is safe to apply them topically. Once applied to the skin, it penetrates quickly into the pores, moves swiftly through the cells into the bloodstream and then throughout the body for maximum internal benefit.

For instance, if you apply essential oil onto the feet, the oil will get to every cell in the body within 21 minutes. If you had a fungus infection in a finger or toe nail, the oil will penetrate it for treatment. What this also means is that topical application of essential oils could provide quick benefit to the specific area of application.

Do not wash essential oils off your body too soon because the longer they stay, the higher the possibility of being absorbed onto the skin. Do not forget to dilute them with carrier oil in most cases so as to provide protection against possible skin sensitivities.

Key areas of application on the body are: Crown of head, Forehead, Temples Behind ears, Upper back, Neck, Abdomen, Soles and top of feet and Ankles.

Applying Essential Oils Topically

1. Tip the oil bottle carefully and drop 2 to 3 drops directly on the desired application area or in the palm of the hand.

2. If applying to the desired area directly, massage the oil onto the desired point of application. If dropping oil in your hand, rub your palms together clockwise and then massage into the skin in a circular motion. Repeat if desired

2. Inhalation

The inhalation of essential oils intensifies the senses and triggers various desired responses in the body. When a person inhales an essential oil, the oil enters the nose and moves straight to the linings of the lungs. It is immediately absorbed into the bloodstream.

There are several methods of inhaling essential oils:

• Direct inhalation – this simply means smelling the essential oils directly. There are of two kinds: basic and steam inhalation. In basic, you drop a little essential oil on a tissue, place it under your nose and inhale. Steam inhalation entails boiling 1 cup of water, adding 3 to 7 drops of your desired oil into it, leaning over the bowl and then breathing in deeply and slowly.

Steam inhalation works very well for colds and chest- related problems. It can be used for its therapeutic benefits day or night, depending upon the blend. However, stop immediately if it causes irritation in your body.

• **Indirect Inhalation**– this can be done through a diffuser whish disperses the essential oil into the air. Certain essential oils can be very stimulating, calming and soothing when diffused in the air. Besides emotional benefits, diffusing essential oils purifies air of unwanted odors and help to reduce the amount of airborne chemicals.

• Another way is through a humidifier. First, you fill it water. Sprinkle 2-6 drops of oil on a small cloth or tissue and then place it in front of the steam emerging from the humidifier.

However, do not put the oil in your humidifier because it will not rise with the water but merely float on top of it. Your humidifier may even be damaged in the process.

3. **Internal Consumption**

Ideally, topical application and inhalation should be sufficient to address almost all issues of concern. Nevertheless, if you must ingest essential oils, be sure to use only those that have been certified safe and labeled as dietary supplements and be sure to follow the stipulated dosage on individual product labels. You should also seek the counsel of a health professional.

Here are a few suggestions of how to take essential oils internally:

• Get an empty capsule, put several oil drops into it and then swallow with water.

• Add 1 to 2 drops to a glass of water or milk.

• Add 1 to 2 drops to your meals when cooking or to a piece of bread.

Some essential oils are also commonly used as flavorings for food products. Peppermint-flavored toothpastes, some flavored soft drinks and certain types of mouthwashes are common examples.

Most Popular Uses For Essential Oils

<u>In the Bath</u>

In this most popular method of enjoying the therapeutic benefit of essential oil, you add a few drops of your preferred essential oil in a heated bath water and then get soaked in it. This way, the oils absorb into your skin and the vapor is inhaled in the process

This is a simple and relaxing method. The only disadvantage is that some oils may stick to the sides of the bath tub thereby lessening the quantity of absorption into your skin. However, you could rub the oils on your body before entering the bath tub to reduce the risk of waste.

<u>Massage</u>

Essentials oils are also applied to the skin through massage. This could be a full body massage or a localized one. The full body massage involves mixing about six drops of oil with your preferred lotion and applying to the skin through repeated rubbing.

Localized massages are applied to specific areas that are causing pain or discomfort such as stiff joints or muscle sprains. The oils are often diluted with carrier oil (about 1 teaspoon carrier oil per about 10 drops essential oils). Facial massages must be carefully conducted so the oils do not get into the eyes, nose or mouth. They require little amount of oils as well.

<u>Fragrancers & Diffusers</u>

A third most popular method of essential oils application is through diffusion which could either be via steam, mist, dry heat or even with the help of fan.

This method is often used to enhance moods, calm the environment and benefit from the therapeutic effects of the oils through inhalation.

The two common types of fragrancers are the standard fragrance and the electrical fragrance. The standard type involves adding essential oils to a bowl of water which is then heated gently to a tea light candle. This process though cheap is not entirely safe due to the exposed flame. For the electric type, the oils are dripped onto a metal plate surface and heated by an electrical part. While this method is safer, the effectiveness of the oils may be damaged if the electrical heat is too strong.

There are many different types of diffusers and nebulizers available that do a great job.

CHAPTER 2

Top Essential Oils For Every Beginner

Lavender

Lavender is known as the Universal Essential Oil because it performs a multitude of functions. It is exceptionally soothing on the skin and produces powerful physical and emotional impact with a scent so relaxing and cooling on the body. It boosts vitality and stamina.

It is also anti-inflammatory, anti-bacterial and anti-depressant, mixing well with a lot of other essential oils. This is the main reason why it is a top choice ingredient for homemade cosmetics and beauty products such as lotions, soaps, gels and creams.

To benefit from its calming and relaxing properties, drop a few drops of lavender oil on your palm (2-3 drops), rub both hands together and then cup over your nose and inhale. You will soon begin to feel the relaxing effect on your mind and body particularly if you have had a bad day. You can also rub on your feet, wrist and ON your ears. Do same for a fussy child.

Do you have rash, burns, acne, scars, wound or any kind of skin trouble? Apply Lavender. You may apply undiluted but if the area is really large, you should mix with carrier oil and apply. To soothe aches and pains, combine 10 drops of essential oil and 2 tablespoons of carrier oil or lotion and then massage areas of discomfort.

Lavender essential oil is effective for hair care and proven to be exceptionally destructive to lice, nits and lice eggs. It controls dandruff, keeps the hair shiny and stimulates the scalp. It also stops hair loss and adds nutrients to the hair.

You can also make your home refreshingly inviting by simmering dried lavender with some citrus peels in a pot of water and let the relaxing fragrance fill your home. Ward off moths in your drawers and closets by placing dried lavender sachets.

Lavender essential oil works wonders for tired and sore muscles. Simply add 4 drops to ½ cup of Epsom salts and soak your cares away. Do not forget to rinse off afterwards. Relieve a stuffy nose by adding 5 drops of lavender to a humidifier.

Massage gently onto the abdomen for menstrual discomfort and if you are concerned your kids may have picked up some germs at play, put a few drops in a roll on bottle and rub gently on the bottoms of their feet for immune support. Alleviate insomnia and enjoy a deep and restful sleep by putting 1-2 drop on the bottoms of your feet or on your pillow before bed time. Repel mosquitoes by adding 2-3 drops lavender to a carrier oil and then spritz on your body.

Overall, a bottle of Lavender is your home will do a whole lot for everyone, including pets as the oil also works well on dogs, cats and horses. It is also gentle enough for a baby's use (dilute 75%). It is an essential oil that will uplifts your spirits and relive your senses.

Lemon
Lemon has various uses to enhance your mood, body and home. A naturally detoxifying substance, lemon essential oil is a cleaning powerhouse.

Simply add a few drops to your cleaning water and you get a complete and safe disinfectant. If you are travelling and you are unsure of the quality of water before you, lemon essential oil is particularly valuable. Add 1drop of Lemon to your water to purify it.

Get rid of any germ you may have come in contact with through sick people, door handles and the likes by putting a drop of Lemon essential oil in your hand and rubbing it around. You are guaranteed of protection from any exposure to germs.

In addition, sticky, gooey residues and price tags can be eliminated by the simple act of adding a drop of lemon oil to it. It will slide off with ease. Cleanse bacteria residue and erase harsh odors on your cutting board by adding a few drops of lemon oil to it. To remove badly burned food in pan, add lemon oil to boiling water and pour on the burnt stuff. Make those smelly shoes fresh again by adding a few drops in them and leaving overnight.

Lemon elevates mood. Simply diffuse to liven up your mood and make your environment fresh, clean and bright. Diffuse in a sick room as well so people around it wouldn't fall ill and the sick person will have a more pleasant disposition. Let the sunshine in!

Lemon essential oil works wonderfully on the skin which is why is usually incorporated into cleansers and scrubs as a natural skin cleanser. It softens skin calluses when it is applied on a callus twice a day.

Lemon essential oil also helps to relieve ear pain and supports the lymphatic system. It deals with respiratory problems like coughs and cold, helping to effectively curb them.

In short, a few drops of lemon added to a whole lot of things will do wonders. For example, to make your hair appear shinier, add a few drops of lemon to your shampoo. To cure bad breath, add a few drops to a teaspoon of honey with warm water and gargle. To help lessen the appearance of cellulite, place a few drops into coconut oil (unrefined) and apply on it.

However, lemon is a type of citrus oil so it has a short shelf life. Do not store for long. If you apply it to skin, keep away from direct sunlight for 48 hours so you don't get skin discoloration. Simply cover with clothes and you will be fine.

Peppermint
All through history, peppermint essential oil has been used to soothe tummy troubles, cure bad breath and relieve headaches, colic, gas and heartburn. Emotionally, peppermint helps to ease depression, eliminate fatigue and soften anger.

By making a peppermint tea, you can soothe sore throat and alleviate indigestion. Simply add 1 drop of peppermint to a ½ cup of hot water, add 1 teaspoon of honey to it, stir and drink. Are you nauseous or experiencing stomach troubles? Add 3-4 drops of Peppermint essential oil to 1 tbsp of carrier oil and rub gently round the tummy.

Do you have a fever? Just add 1 to 2 drops of peppermint to a bowl of cool water. Get a clean cloth, dip it in and then sponge down (keep away from the eyes). Alternatively, apply a few drops gently to the bottoms of your feet.

Peppermint oil is highly effective for headaches. Combine 1to 2 peppermint essential oil and carrier oil and then applying to your temples (again, avoid the eyes!) and along the back of your neck. Finally, cup your hands and inhale. This helps to cleanse the sinuses as well.

To keep your energy up, apply a few drops to your shoulders and back of neck throughout the day and inhale to boost your mood and reduce fatigue, especially before and after workouts. Diffuse to enhance focus while studying in your room.

Give yourself a pedicure and add to your beauty routine. If your feet are tired from a long day, this stuff is amazing for the bottoms of your feet.

If you get sunburned, treat it like you will do for the fever. However, if your skin is too sensitive for the cloth, get a small spritzer bottle and then spray the Peppermint water on your skin, avoiding the eyes.

Are your muscles aching from overwork or exercises? Mix 2 drops peppermint in carrier oil. Rub it down on those aching muscles.

Get rid of those mice and ants in your pantry by doing this: put some peppermint in cotton balls and stuff them where the rodents and insects are coming in. A natural spider repellent, peppermint oil diffused into the air will send those spiders running. To kill aphids, mix 4 to 5 drops in a bottle of water and spray on plants.

However, peppermint isn't safe for children under 5 years of age. Also, it should always be diluted.

Sandalwood

A powerful fighter of bacteria and viruses, sandalwood essential oil, offers a host of benefits to the skin when properly applied. Let's consider a few of these applications.

To fight rashes, itchiness or inflammation, combine 3-7 drops of sandalwood, one teaspoon of lime juice and one teaspoon of turmeric powder. Apply thinly to the skin and leave for 20- 30 minutes. Rinse with cool water and pat gently to dry. Redness or swelling may take time to subside but itchiness should quickly fade.

Sandalwood helps to even skin tone so if you have uneven tans, mix 7-10 drops of sandalwood with five teaspoons of coconut oil and two teaspoons of jojoba oil. Massage this blend into overexposed areas.

For pimples and acne, combine 3 to 7 drops of sandalwood essential oil, one teaspoon of spring water or rosewater and one teaspoon of turmeric powder. Apply thinly to the skin and leave for about thirty minutes. Rinse face with lukewarm water and gently dry. Do this one or two times daily and noticeable changes will be observed after only 48 hours.

An excellent moisturizer, sandalwood can aid dry skin. For specific areas, just apply 1-2 diluted drops to skin and massage. For a full body application, dilute with a carrier oil like jojoba oil and your skin will feel soft and hydrated.

To treat bug bite, mix 5 to 7 drops of sandalwood with one teaspoon of lavender oil, one teaspoon of turmeric and just enough water for a paste. Apply this paste to the bug bite immediately to reduce swelling and stop itching.

In addition, sandalwood oil is helpful for respiratory problems via steam inhalation. It is also great for conditioning dry hair. Simply apply 4-6 drops of it to your hair after a shower and your hair will be moisturized, soft and shiny.

Tea Tree

Also called Melaleuca, tea tree oil can be applied to the skin either undiluted (neat) or diluted. If you have sensitive skin or if using with kids, dilute in a carrier oil before use.

Tea tree is analgesic which means that it reduces pain. For a toothache, mix 1 drop of tea tree oil in 4 oz of warm water and swish around in the mouth 3-4 times per day but DO NOT SWALLOW. For ear infections, rub 1-2 drops all around the base of the ear every 2 to3 hours.

As a powerful antifungal, tea tree fights ringworm, Candida and other fungal skin infections. To address these, dilute 5-6 drops in a tablespoon of coconut oil and rub onto the infection 3-4 times a day. (For yeast infections, do not use in the genital area because it can burn really badly)

Other skin issues like acne can be cleared up faster by rubbing a drop of this oil onto problem areas 2 to3 times daily. Also apply tea tree essential oil undiluted to the feet for Athlete's Foot or blend5-6 drops with 1 tablespoon of coconut oil and massage feet before bed time and when you wake up.

For Canker Sores/Cold Sores, mix 1-2 drops in 1 teaspoon of a carrier oil and dab onto the sore as many times as possible during the day. Make the same blend for eczema but massage onto the affected area.

Warts are tough to eliminate so apply tea tree neat as many times as possible all through the day until the warts vanishes.

CHAPTER 3

Recipes For Body & Skin Care

Face Blend For Normal Skin

2 drops Lavender essential oil

1 drop Geranium essential oil

1 tablespoon Sweet Almond Oil

Instructions

Blend oils and use on face after cleaning and toning.

Face Blend For Dry Skin

1 drop Roman Chamomile essential oil

2 drops Neroli essential oil

1 tbsp Sweet Almond Oil

Instructions

Blend oils and use on face as needed.

Face Blend for Mature Skin

2 drops Frankincense essential oil

1 drop Rose essential oil

1 tbsp carrier oil of choice

Instructions

Blend oils and use on face to rejuvenate and tone mature skin.

Skin Toner

1 drop Rosewood essential oil

1 drop Palmarosa essential oil

2 drops Lavender essential oil

8 oz Distilled water

Instructions

1. Pour distilled water and then essentials oil into a clean bottle, mixing well.

2. After cleansing, apply the toner to your skin with a cotton ball. Shake well before use.

Sunburn Relief

60 drops Lavender essential oil

25 drops Helichrysum essential oil

2 oz Jojoba

2 oz Aloe Vera gel

Instructions

Blend together and store in a cool place. Apply as needed.

Lotion Blend For Cracked Skin

1 ounce unscented Lotion

10 drops Lavender essential oil

5 drops Neroli essential oil

5 drops Helichrysum essential oil

Instructions

1. Mix the essentials oils together and add to lotion.

2. Apply several times in a day to stimulate healing of the cracks and to regenerate new cells.

Antiwrinkle Oil

10 drops Lavender essential oil

10 drops Neroli essential oil

10 drops Rosehip seed essential oil

10 drops Frankincense essential oil

10 drops Carrotseed essential oil

10 drops Fennel essential oil

2 drops Rosemary essential oil

3 drops Lemon essential oil

2 tablespoons Apricot Kernel, Hazelnut or Sweet almond

Instructions

1. Blend all the ingredients in a bottle.

2. Apply 3-4 drops to the face and neck area every night after cleansing & toning the skin.

Dry Skin Formula

25 drops Carrotseed essential oil

6 drops Sandalwood essential oil

2 drops Geranium essential oil

4 drops Neroli essential oil

1 teaspoon Camellia oil

1 teaspoon Jojoba

Sesame oil - 1 teaspoon

Instructions

1. Blend all the ingredients in a 1 oz bottle, shaking thoroughly to mix.

2. Apply 4 to 6 drops of blend two times daily to dry area.

Silky Clay Mask

For all skin types

½ teaspoon kaolin clay

2 drops rose essential oil

1½ teaspoons green clay (preferably French)

1 tablespoon rosewater

1½ tablespoons aloe Vera gel

Instructions:

1. Mix kaolin and green clays together.

2. Add the rosewater, aloe vera gel and oils.

3. Use and refrigerate mixture for 4weeks.

Peppermint Foot Scrub

1 tsp. peppermint essential oil

½ cup jojoba oil

1 cup turbinado sugar

Instructions

1. Combine ingredients well until it forms a paste.

2. Transfer to a glass container and seal.

3. Use within 3 months.

Skin Firming Blend For Flabby Skin

5 drops Cypress EO

5 drops Geranium EO

8 drops Patchouli EO

1 drop Sandalwood EO

1/2 teaspoon Jojoba oil

Instructions

Combine well and massage affected areas before going to bed and occasionally in the mornings.

Strawberry or Raspberry Body Rub

3 ripe strawberries or raspberries

3-4 drops Lemon or Lavender essential oil

1 tbsp almond or apricot oil

1 cup fine sea salt

Instructions

1. Pour salt into a bowl.

2. Add the raspberries or strawberries and essential oil and then mash together.

3. Rub a small handful of this mixture over your body gentle circular motions, emphasizing your elbows, knees and heels. Rinse off.

4. No need to apply moisturizer. Store covered in refrigerator for 2 weeks

Purse –Size After Sun Spray

15 ml Glass Spray Bottle

2 drops Lavender essential oil

2 drops Roman chamomile essential oil

2 drops Melaleuca esssential oil

1 tbsp Fractionated Coconut oil

1/4 tsp vitamin E oil

1/4 cup Aloe Vera Juice

Instructions

1. Combine all ingredients in glass spray bottle, putting the oils first and filling with the Aloe Vera Juice

2. Shake thoroughly to incorporate ingredients.

3. Spray as needed onto skin to improve skin tone.

Revitalizing Neck Gel

15 drops Peppermint EO

2 oz Aloe Vera Gel (unscented)

Instructions:

1. Combine ingredients in a small jar until it appears cloudy.

2. Apply a little quantity to the back of your neck, massaging gently.

Citrus Coffee Body Scrub

1-3 drops lemon essential oil

1-3 drops orange essential oil

1 cup coconut oil, melted

½ cup coconut sugar

1 cup coffee grounds

Instructions

1. Combine ingredients well in a bowl.

2. Keep blend at room temperature and then use.

3. Store any leftover in a mason jar

Soothing Foot Lotion

20 drops eucalyptus essential oil

20 drops peppermint essential oil

10 drops tea tree essential oil

1 tbsp sweet almond

1 tsp Vitamin E Oil

1 cup lotion base

Instructions:

1. Combine all ingredients thoroughly

2. Stir well and transfer to a glass container.

EO for Bags Under Eyes

1 drop Lavender essential oil

1 drop Roman Chamomile essential oil

30mls Aloe Vera gel or lotion/cream

Instructions:

1. Combine essential oils with aloe Vera gel or lotion/ cream, mixing well.

2. Cleanse and dry face daily and then rub the blend gently below and above the eye socket.

3. be careful so you don't get the blend into your eyes.

Recipes For Skin & Body Treatment

Aromatherapy Treatment For Acne

10 drops Lavender essential oil

3 drops Geranium essential oil

7 drops Tea Tree or Lemongrass essential oil

30ml Aloe Vera gel

Instructions:

1. Mix all ingredients well in a dark glass bottle.

2. Apply a small amount to areas of the skin twice daily. Avoid nose, lips and eyes.

3. Noticeable result after constant use within a few weeks.

Dermatitis Treatment

3 drops Melaleuca essential oil

5 drops Myrrh essential oil

10 drops Lavender essential oil

5 drops Helichrysum essential oil

1 teaspoon extra virgin coconut oil

Instructions:

Mix together and apply topically on affected area daily.

Eczema Relief Roller Blend

15 drops Melaleuca essential oil

15 drops Helichrysum essential oil

40 drops Lavender essential oil

Instructions:

1. Mix ingredients in a 10ml roller bottle and add to fractionated coconut oil.

2. Apply to affected area.

Steam Bath For Acne & Oily Skin

6 drops Juniper Berry essential oil

4 drops Lemon essential oil

4 drops Cypress essential oil

Instructions

1. Combine oils in bowl of very hot water and carry out the steam inhalation.

2. Rinse face after 5-10 minutes with cool water and pat dry.

Athletes Foot Relief Oil

6 drops Myrrh essential oil

8 drops Eucalyptus essential oil

10 drops Tea Tree essential oil

6 drops Thyme essential oil

2 oz carrier oil of choice

Instructions

1. Blend together in a clean container. Apply a few drops to affected area directly. Do this 1-2 times daily.

2. Noticeable relief within 1-2 days.

Ringworm Treatment

30 drops Lavender essential oil

30 drops Melaleuca essential oil

30 drops Thyme essential oil

Instructions:

Combine all and apply 2-3 drops topically on infected area 3 times a day for 10- 12 days

Eczema/ lubricant Recipe

12 drops lavender essential oil

20 drops evening primrose oil

12 drops roman chamomile essential oil

4 oz jojoba oil

Instructions:

1. Combine all and apply to affected areas. Alternatively, use it as a daily skin lubricant.

3. This recipe is effective and gentle on children with eczema.

Lice & Scabies External Body Treatment

2 drops Cinnamon essential oil

2 drops Pine essential oil

2 drops Rosemary essential oil

1 drop Thyme essential oil

5 ml Carrier oil

Instructions:

Combine and apply on affected area directly.

Corn And Callus Blend

12 drops Lavender essential oil

6 drops Myrrh essential oil

2 oz Sweet almond

Instructions

1. Combine all in bottle, shaking well to mix.

2. Massage into the affected area daily to soften calluses and corns.

Warts Eliminator

12 drops Lemon essential oil

4 drops Tea Tree essential oil

4 drops Thyme essential oil

3 drops Cypress essential oil

4 drops Bergamot FCF essential oil

1 tbsp Jojoba oil or 2 tbsp jojoba if using on kids and the elderly

Instructions:

1. Mix together all ingredients in a bottle.

2. Apply 2 drops of mixture to wart and then cover with a Band-Aid.

3. Apply daily for 2 weeks.

CHAPTER 4

Recipes For Hair Care

For Oily Hair

2 tbsp Grapeseed essential oil

9 drops Ylang Ylang essential oil

9 drops Lime essential oil

8 drops Rosemary essential oil

Instructions

1. Combine, shake well and apply a tsp to hair and scalp, massaging in.

2. Let it penetrate overnight or for several hours.

3. Wash hair with a natural unscented shampoo twice.

4. Use thrice a week.

Hair Loss Recipe

1 tbsp Jojoba oil

1 tbsp Sweet almond oil

10 drops Lavender EO

40 drops Carrotseed EO

6 drops Clary Sage EO

4 drops Rosemary EO

4 drops Roman Chamomile EO

<u>Instructions</u>

1. Combine, shake well and apply a few drops to scalp, massaging in.

2. Leave until absorbed in. Apply many times in a week.

Mild Hair Loss Remedy

<u>Instructions</u>

1. Add 1 - 2 drops Rosemary essential oil to your shampoo

2. Use it daily to stimulate hair follicle.

Hair Moisturizer

1 ounce Jojoba

8 drops Cedarwood essential oil

8 drops Lavender essential oil

12 drops Rosemary essential oil

<u>Instructions</u>

1. Combine in a PET plastic bottle, shake well and apply a tsp to hair and scalp, massaging in.

2. Put a shower cap on and wrap with towel. Let it sit for 15- 20 minutes.

3. Shampoo and rinse hair twice. Dry and style hair as normal.

4. Carry out weekly or monthly.

Dandruff & Scaly Scalp Blend

2 drops Atlas cedarwood essential oil

2 drops Rosemary essential oil

2 drops tea tree oil essential oil

2 drops Lavender essential oil

1/2 ounce Jojoba

Instructions

Combine and apply to scalp

Hair Growth/ Softener Recipe

2 drops Thyme essential oil

3 drops Rosemary essential oil

2 drops Cedar essential oil

1 ounce Grapeseed

1 tbsp Jojoba

Instructions

1. Combine ingredients into a tight bottle.

2. Massage into your scalp every night.

3. Rinse the next morning in cool water and shampoo.

3. Use thrice a week for oily hair and once for normal.

Wood Haven Beard Oil

Oil and beautify your beard, moisturize the dry skin underneath it and smell really wonderful!

3 drops peppermint essential oil

1/4oz sweet almond oil

5 drops tea tree oil essential oil

3/4oz jojoba oil

Instructions

1. Combine in 1 oz bottle, shake well, dap on your fingers and rub on your beards.

2. Best use after a shower when your beard is washed and your skin is fresh.

Minty Fresh Beard Oil

1/2oz sweet almond oil

2 drops tea tree oil

5 drops peppermint oil

2 drops orange oil

1/2oz jojoba oil

3/4oz jojoba oil

Instructions

1. Combine in 1 oz bottle, shake well, dap on your fingers and rub on your beards.

2. Best use after a shower when your beard is washed and your skin is fresh.

Fall Face Foliage Beard Oil

3/4oz sweet almond oil

2 drops tea tree oil

2 drops cinnamon cassia oil

2 drops orange oil

1/4oz jojoba oil

<u>Instructions</u>

1. Combine in 1 oz bottle, shake well, dap on your fingers and rub on your beards.

2. Best use after a shower when your beard is washed and your skin is fresh.

CHAPTER 5

Recipes For Emotional Well Being

Certain essential oil blends help to balance our moods and energize our bodies and spirit. Many of them can be created easily. One of the most pleasurable mode of application is to use them in your bath.

<u>Simple Blends</u>

Combine these blends with a tablespoon of apricot or almond oil and massage over your body. Alternatively rub 2-3 drops on your chest and shower before going to work.

Anti- Anger Blend

2 drops Patchouli

3 drops Orange

Anti- Fear Blend

2 drops Bergamot

3 drops Grapefruit

Confidence Booster Blend

2 drops Rosemary

3 drops Orange

Memory Enhancing blend

2 drops Lemon

3 drops Rosemary

Stress Relieving Blend

3 drops Clary Sage

1 drop Lavender

1 drop Lemon

Revitalizing Oil Bath

12 drops Geranium essential oil

6 drops Lemon essential oil

6 drops Sandalwood essential oil

2 drops Clary Sage essential oil

4tbs Jojoba, Almond Castor, or Sunflower carrier oil

Instructions

1. Pour carrier oil into a glass bottle and then add essential oils.

2. Cover and shake thoroughly and store for 2 weeks in a dark place

3. Once matured, add 1 tbsp of the scented oil to the bath tub.

5. Swish and enjoy your revitalizing bath.

Liquid Sleep Blend

7 drops Vetiver essential oil

20 drops Lavender essential oil

Instructions

1. Combine in a 1/3 oz (approx. 10 ml) roller bottle.

2. Top with Fractionated coconut Oil

3. Apply to bottoms of feet before bedtime.

Anxiety Roller Blend

12 drops Ginger essential oil

6 drops Ylang Ylang essential oil

9 drops Lavender essential oil

9 drops Sandalwood essential oil

Instructions

1. Combine in a roller bottle.

2. Top with Fractionated coconut Oil in a 10ml bottle.

Quiet Mind

For neurological issues and anxieties

20 drops Vetiver

5 drops Frankincese

20 drops Whisper

4 drops Bergamot

Instructions

1. Combine in a roller bottle and fill with Fractionated Coconut Oil.

2. Shake and apply to base of skull, spine, bottom of feet or wrists.

Blissful/Happy Oil Bath

10 drops Sandalwood

5 drops Jasmine

5 drops Rose

5 drops Bergamot

4tbsp Jojoba, Almond Castor, or Sunflower carrier oil

Instructions

1. Pour carrier oil into a glass bottle and then add essential oils.

2. Cover and shake thoroughly and store for 2 weeks in a dark place

3. Once matured, add 1 tbsp of the scented oil to the bath tub.

5. Swish and enjoy your bath. Remain happy!

Sensuous Oil Bath

20 drops Jasmine

8 drops Orange

4tbsp Jojoba, Almond Castor, or Sunflower carrier oil

Instructions

1. Pour carrier oil into a glass bottle and then add essential oils.

2. Cover and shake thoroughly and store for 2 weeks in a dark place

3. Once matured, add 1 tbsp of the scented oil to the bath tub.

5. Swish and enjoy your sensual bath. Remain happy!

Relaxing Oil Bath

12 drops Sandalwood essential oil

8 drops Orange essential oil

4 drops Rose essential oil

2 drops Pine essential oil

2 drops Lemon essential oil

4tbsp Jojoba, Almond Castor, or Sunflower carrier oil

Instructions

1. Pour carrier oil into a glass bottle and then add essential oils.

2. Cover and shake thoroughly and store for 2 weeks in a dark place

3. Once matured, add 1 tbsp of the scented oil to the bath tub.

5. Swish and enjoy your anti-stress and depression relaxing bath.

CHAPTER 6

Recipes For Household

Everyone should replace disinfectants with natural cleansers as studies have proven that store-bought cleaners are toxic and can make you ill. What better way to do this than with all natural essential oils. They are the cheapest and safest cleaning agent, helping to kill germs and bacteria and to naturally freshen up.

Essential Oils clean by…

- Deodorizing
- Disinfecting
- Eliminating Mold
- Eliminating Mildew

Another wonderful thing about essential oils is the natural fragrance it gives to your home all day long. The scent from aromatherapy oils is so strong that they can make the best air fresheners in your home. This is also good for your pets.

Lavender/ Tea Tree Spray Cleaner

3 drops Tea Tree essential oil

1/4 tsp Lavender essential oil

1 tsp borax

2 tbsp white vinegar

2 cups hot water

Instructions

1. Mix together all the ingredients and stir until completely dissolve.

2. Pour mixture into spray bottle.

3. Spray as needed on surfaces except glass.

4. Scrub and then rinse with a clean and damp, cloth.

Heavy Duty Toilet Formula

5 drops lemon essential oil

1 cup white vinegar

10 drops lavender essential oil

3/4 cup borax

Instructions

1. Combine ingredients in a squirt bottle.

2. Flush to wet the inside of the bowl and then pour mixture into the toilet bowl.

3. Let it sit unused for several hours. Scrub bowl and flush toilet to rinse.

Tea Tree Toilet Bowl Scrub

½ teaspoon tea tree essential oil

1 cup distilled white vinegar

½ cup baking soda

Instructions

1. Combine essential oil and vinegar in a small spray bottle.

2. Spray the mixture inside the bowl, lid, handle and toilet seat.

3. Let it sit for several minutes.

3. Sprinkle the baking soda inside toilet bowl and the scrub inside of bowl using a toilet brush.

4. Wipe vinegar solution off seat, lid, and handle with a clean dry cloth.

Homemade All-Purpose Cleaner

20 lemon or grapefruit essential oil

2 teaspoons castile soap

1 cup water

Instructions

1. Combine ingredients in a spray bottle.

2. Shake well before use.

Tub &Shower Scrub

Prevent and remove mold and mildew buildup with this recipe.

10 drops Lavender essential oil

10 drops Tea Tree essential oil

10 drops Geranium essential oil

1/2 Cup Baking Soda

Instructions

1. Combine all ingredients. Use a damp cloth or sponge to scrub shower and/or bathtub.

2. For areas with serious mildew buildup, mix water and 20 drops of Tea Tree together in a spray bottle and then spray area daily for 5 days and afterwards 2 times weekly.

Carpet Refresher

7-10 drops of essential oil of choice

1 cup cornstarch or baking soda

<u>Instructions</u>

1. Combine ingredients in a large bowl.

2. Use a fork to break any clumps up and stir thoroughly.

3. Pour the mixture into a cheese shaker. Sprinkle generously over the carpet.

4. Wait for 30 minutes and then vacuum.

Dishwashing Liquid

Not suited for automatic dishwashers.

10 drops Orange essential oil

10 drops Lavender essential oil

10 drops Lemon essential oil

Liquid castile soap

<u>Instructions</u>

1. Put the liquid soap in a 32oz. squirt bottle, filling it up.

2. Add the oils and then shake well.

Kitchen Sink Scrub

1/8 Cup Vinegar

1/2 Cup Baking Soda

5 drops Orange essential oil

5 drops Lemon essential oil

Instructions

1. Combine all the ingredients

2. Try Bergamot or Lime also.

Combs And Brushes

20 drops eucalyptus, lavender or tea-tree oil

½ cup distilled white vinegar

1½ cups water

Instructions

1. Combine ingredients in a container.

2. Soak brushes and combs for 20 minutes

3. Rinse them and air-dry.

Toilets

2 tsp tea-tree oil

2 cups water

Instructions

1. Combine in a spray bottle. Shake well, then spritz along the toilet's inner rim.

2. Let it sit for 30 minutes then scrub.

3. Alternatively, place a few drops of your preferred essential oil on the inside of the toilet-paper tube. This will release the scent every time the paper is used.

Scuffed Floors

1. Apply 2-4 drops tea-tree oil to the spots.

2. Wipe the excess oil with a cloth and then rub in distilled white vinegar.

Windows

10 drops lemongrass essential oil

2 ounces water

Instructions

1. Combine and use to wipe grime off your windows.

2. This repels flies as well.

Fire Logs

1. Place 1 drop sandalwood, cypress, cedar wood or pine essential oil on fire log.

2. Wait for 30 minutes then burn fire log.

3. Use only 1 perfume log at a time as a little goes a long way.

Stuffed Animals

1. Place a few drops of chamomile or lavender on a stuffed animal.

2. Place in a plastic bag and leave overnight.

3. The next day, the stuff animal will wear a dispersed fragrant that will soothe kids and others.

4. This can last for about 2 weeks.

Citrus Glass Shiner

1 tablespoon borax

4 oz water

4 oz apple cider vinegar

1 tbsp orange essential oil

1 tbsp lemon essential oil

Instructions

1. Combine all the ingredients in a plastic spray bottle.

2. Shake well before use.

Spicy Orange Air Freshener

2 drops Cinnamon Leaf

5 drops Orange

4 oz. distilled water

Instructions

1. Pour the distilled water in a spray bottle and add the essential oils to it, shaking well.

2. Spray as needed.

Citrus Air Freshener

50 drops Lemon Essential Oil

10 drops Red Mandarin

50 drops Pink Grapefruit

10 drops Patchouli

4 oz. Pure Water

Instructions

1. Pour the pure water into a mist spray bottle. Add essential oils, tighten cap and shake thoroughly.

2. Spray into the air. Scent will become stronger as the mist ages in the bottle.

CHAPTER 7

Other Essential Oil Recipes

Beauty, Aromatherapy, Pets And More

Foot Deodorizing Powder

2 drops Sage essential oil

2 drops Spearmint essential oil

2 drops Coriander essential oil

2 ounce Talc Powder

1 tablespoon Baking soda

Instructions

1. Add the baking soda to bottle of talc powder, shaking.

2. Add the essential oils to a ball or cotton pad and drop inside the baking soda/ talc bottle.

3. Shake thoroughly and leave for a 2-4 days before using.

4. Apply to your feet and also inside your shoes.

Simple Deodorant Stick

1/4 cup cornstarch

1/4 cup baking soda

1/4 cup coconut oil

10-20 drops essential oil of choice

Instructions

1. Combine all using a stand mixer or hand.

2. Pack into deodorant containers. This makes 2 sticks

Softening Lip Balm

6 drops Spearmint, Orange, lime or Peppermint essential oil

4 tbsp apricot oil

2 tsp grated beeswax

1 tsp Shea butter

1 tsp carrot infused oil

Instructions

1. Add the Shea butter, beeswax and apricot oil to a glass Pyrex jug. Let it stay in a fry pan of simmering water and then melt ingredients together.

2. Add the carrot infused oil, blend well and once cool, add the essential oil.

3. Pour into small d glass jars. Cover tightly, label and date product.

Homemade Aftershave

15 drops Coriander oil

20 drops Orange oil

10 drops Cinnamon oil

3 tablespoons alcohol

2 tablespoon witch hazel

2 tablespoons distilled water

1 tablespoon glycerin

10 drops Bay oil

Instructions

1. Add 1 tablespoon alcohol to a small mixing jug then add the essential oil drops, mixing well.

2. In another mixing jug, add the remaining alcohol, distilled water, witch hazel and then the glycerin, mixing well.

3. Add the essential oil/alcohol mixture to the other mixture, very slowly stirring continuously.

4. Pour into a dark, glass bottle, sealing tightly. Store it for 1-2 weeks in a cool, dark place.

5. After 1 or 2 weeks, filter the mixture through filter paper then dispense into a clean container.

6. Splash aftershave on the face after shaving.

Lavender/Tea Tree Blemish Remover

10 drops tea tree essential oil

10 drops lavender essential oil

3 drops lemon essential oil

5 drops rosemary essential oil

1 ounce jojoba oil

Instructions

1. Fill a 1 oz small bottle with jojoba oil.

2. Add the essential oils, cover bottle and shake well.

Lavender & Lemon Solid Perfume

5 drop rosemary essential oil

15 drops lavender essential oil

3 drops lemongrass essential oil

3g beeswax

12g sweet almond oil

Instructions

1. Melt the beeswax and sweet almond oil together in a small pan over low heat.

2. Remove and let it cool for 1 minute. Add the essential oils and mix.

3. Decant into 1/4 oz tins. This fills 2 tins.

Elbow Soft Cream

2 drops Carrot essential oil

4 drops Lavender essential oil

3 drops Orange essential oil

½ teaspoon vitamin E oil

1 tbsp grated beeswax

1 tbsp rose water

¼ cup cocoa butter

¼ cup avocado oil

Instructions

1. Add the avocado oil, cocoa butter and beeswax to a glass Pyrex jug. Place jug in a fry pan of simmering water to melt ingredients.

2. To another Pyrex jug, add the rose water and place also in the fry pan of simmering water.

3. Once melted, add the vitamin E oil and mix well.

4. Add the rose water per drop to the wax/ oil mixture. After adding about a tablespoon remove from the heat and keep adding the rose water slowly and mixing with a small whisk.

5. Once mixture begins to thicken, add the essential oils and mix.

6. Divide cream into sterilized glass jars. Cover tightly, label and date product.

Foaming Face Wash

1/3 cup castile soap

10 drops Ylang Ylang essential oil

4 drops Lemongrass essential oil

6 drops Patchouli essential oil

2/3 cup distilled or filtered water

1/2 tsp sweet almond oil

Instructions

1. Pour the sweet almond oil and castile soap into a foaming soap dispenser.

2. Add the essential oils and swirl.

3. Fill the container with water and screw. Use every day for radiant skin!

Fresh Feet Bath

3 drops Geranium oil

4 drops Lime oil

2 drops Lemongrass oil

Instructions

1. Fill a foot spa or tub o with warm water and then add the essential oils.

2. Soak feet for up to 10 minutes. Dry thoroughly.

Aromatherapy

Feet Therapy For Cold & Chilly Feelings

6 drops Geranium essential oil

4 drops Rosemary essential oil

10 drops Lemon essential oil

Instructions:

1. Combine all in an amber bottle. Add 3-4 drops to a basin of hot (but not so hot) water.

2. Soak feet for 15- 30 minutes. Dry and apply some lotion.

3. Cover feet with socks, slippers or shoes.

Menstrual Cramps Bath Remedy

5 drops Lavender

2 drops Cypress

2 drops Nutmeg

2 drops Peppermint

1/2 cup Epsom and/or sea salt

Instructions:

1. Combine oils and add to bath salts.

2. Soak for 20- 30 min. Rinse and take a rest, elevating your legs.

Allergy Relief

Ease symptoms of seasonal allergies such as stuffy nose, itchy eyes, tight sinuses, dry cough & headaches.

20 drops Lemon essential oil

20 drops Peppermint essential oil

20 drops Lavender essential oil

Instructions:

1. Combine essential oils in first in 10 ml roller bottle.

2. Fill the rest of the roller bottle with Fractionated Coconut Oil

3. Roll on back of neck and rub on hands, inhaling deeply. Also, place directly under bridge of nose.

3. Use as many times as needed for relief.

Cold Feet/Hands Blend

4 drops Black Pepper

2 drops Thyme

Instructions:

1. Combine and fill roller bottle (1/3oz) with fractionated coconut oil

2. Apply before going out in cold temperatures and also when coming back inside.

Wonder Roller Blend

9 drops Cypress essential oil

6 drops Melaleuca essential oil

15 drops Rosemary essential oil

12 drops Eucalyptus essential oil

12 drops Peppermint essential oil

Instructions:

1. Combine essential oils in first in 10 ml roller bottle.

2. Fill the rest of the roller bottle with Fractionated Coconut Oil

3. Apply to the chest to relieve cough. Alternatively add 1 tsp virgin coconut oil and use as rub.

Liver Cleanse With Lemon & Peppermint

1 drop Lemon essential oil

1 drop Peppermint essential oil

1 tsp -1 tbsp fresh lemon juice

Instructions:

Combine and take every morning when out from bed to cleanse those toxins from your body.

Super- Duper Asthma/Coughing Relief

40 drops Peppermint (*opens airways and aids the increase of other oils' absorption*)

50 drops Eucalyptus (*opens airways and sinuses*)

30 drops Lavender (*calms and soothes*)

30 drops Lemon (*cuts down the congestion*)

30 drops Lime (*good for respiratory issues*)

20 drops Rosemary (*helps with congestion, breathing and coughing*)

20 drops Cypress (*helps with coughing and breathing*)

15 drops Frankincense (*helps with everything*)

Instructions

Combine in a 15ml bottle and fill with fractionated coconut oil.

Tea Remedy For Cough

1 drop lemon essential oil

1 drop clove essential oil

1-2 drops honey

8oz water (boiling)

Extra virgin coconut oil carrier (1 tablespoon, optional)

Instructions:

1. Add oils and honey to boiling water. Blend at high speed for 60 seconds.

2. Put a towel over your head, lean over the steaming cup to enjoy the therapeutic steam.

Pet Odor Control Blend

10 drops Lavender

6 drops Lemon

10 drops Geranium

Instructions

1. Fill a 1-oz spray bottle with water and then pour the essential oils into it.

2. Shake well and spray directly on dog.

3. Hold the bottle at least 10 inches away from him and do not spray on head and eyes.

BOOK 2

Essential Oils For Kids And Babies

A Simple Guide To Aromatherapy And Using Essential Oils For Children

Coral Miller

INTRODUCTION

Essential Oils, Aromatherapy And Your Kid

Essential oils are natural aromatic compounds that are found in plants. They are extracted from a large variety of aromatic herbs by steam distillation or cold- pressing. Since they are aromatic compounds of the plants from which they are extracted, they retain all the healing qualities of the mother-herb. Consequently, they are about 70 times more powerful than herbs. Although they are called "oils", they are in fact a liquid and do not feel oily at all. They are highly concentrated, extremely powerful, richly fragrant, safe and without side effects.

Essential oils are used for aromatherapy, which is the art of treating diseases with herbal essences. Aromatherapy dates back thousands of years. The ancient people discovered that aromatic compounds in essential oils have direct effect on their mental, emotional and physical health. This is holistic therapy because it not only aims for the individual's body, but for his mind and soul as well.

Babies are born with clear and beautiful skin. As they grow, they require extra care to sustain their cherubic beauty. Children's beauty tips include an extensive care that starts from skin to health. A lot of children's products such as shampoos, powders and baby wipes contain harmful chemicals. Exposing them to these harsh chemical-based beauty products and medicines is dangerous due to their tender and sensitive skin. Using natural products with essential oils will help to protect your kid's health from these harmful products. Besides good food, plenty of rest, outdoor plays and good hygiene to help kids grow and develop well, there is need to use essential oils to address their internal and external beauty needs.

These little ones must be protected from these harmful products which may have devastating health effect in the long run. Although some reputed brands have included many skin care and health products for children, choosing the right product may be difficult as manufacturers aren't always truthful about their product ingredients' and claims.

Then again, nature has its own tender way of healing and helping the body recover its energy and health. This is the only thing our kids need: a little help for their fight with an intrusive external agent. Therefore, it makes a lot of sense to use essential oil for general wellbeing.

Benefits Of Essential Oils For Kids And Babies

Essential oils provide tremendous benefits physically and emotionally. Since they come from therapeutic plants, they provide a wide range of health benefits. And since they are natural compounds without a single chemical ingredient, they are safer than commercial products, particularly when used correctly. They are affordable and also handy as they can be made quickly, easily and stored. They should be an important part of the natural remedies for every home.

Essential oils help to treat different ailments in kids and even babies. They help relieve a runny nose, get better sleep (due to their calming effect), treat some skin issues like scratches, rushes and minor bruises as well as provide relief from many ailments like fever, constipation, jaundice, hiccoughs, earaches and teething pain.

Where antibiotics cannot penetrate cell membrane, essential oils can penetrate cells to kill bacteria and viruses easily. They penetrate the skin and are quickly absorbed into the body where they fight and kill bacteria and viruses.

Essential oils can also be part of natural ingredients for baby and kids' oils, lotions, powders and wipes. As wonderful additive to natural products, they also provide these products with a unique fragrance due to their aromatic nature.

Using Essential Oils Safely

Before you use essential oils for babies and children, you must exercise some measure of caution. Essential oils are extremely strong and must never be used internally on small children. Also, keep your essential oils out of the reach of babies and small children to prevent the risk of ingestion. However, if ingestion occurs, do not induce vomit but take your child immediately to the emergency ward.

Dilution of the essential oils is very important. Essential oils must always be used diluted in a carrier oil. Virgin Coconut Oil is an excellent carrier oil for babies because it is nutrient-rich but others like sunflower, almond, grape seed and apricot kernel may also be used. Other dilution material like milk, vegetable glycerin or raw honey may also be used.

Using neat (undiluted) essential oils may cause seizures or irritation to the skin. Do not use essential oils on children's face and in and around their noses. Their strong fragrance (especially the ones that contain menthol) may slow their breathing and lead to respiratory problems.

Be careful when using essential oils with babies. They may be allergic to a certain compound as you haven't discovered yet all his/her sensitivities. It is recommended that you introduce no more than an essential oil a day. After that, watch your baby's reaction. If there is an allergy problem, the effects should appear in about 30-40 minutes. The best thing you can do is to initially test a small part of the skin when applying lotions or massage oils.

When using oils with children, more isn't better. Be sure to always dilute well and use only a very small amount of oil as it goes a long way to soothe and calm. A larger quantity may lead to fussiness and agitation.

Safety Tips

Have these safety tips at your fingertips:

* Do not use undiluted essential oil directly on your kid's skin (burning and irritation may occur).
* If essential oils are used in bath, always disperse by using a bath gel or dilute in a water soluble carrier like vegetable glycerin or raw unfiltered honey.
* Avoid getting essential oils in eyes. If you do, flush eyes with milk.
* Do not place undiluted essential oil too close to kid's face.
* Do not use undiluted essential oil in a diffuser as the scent will be too strong for your child.
* Never ever ingest an essential oil. If ingested in error, give liquids such as cream, milk, half and half and immediately call your doctor. A few drops usually isn't life threatening but it is safer to take these precautions.
* Do not use essential oils on premature babies on account of their delicate and almost transparent skin. It is best to wait until the skin has attained more maturity.

Using Essential Oils For Children

There are different ways of using the essential oils for children such as baths, inhalations, compresses, massages and sprays. However, the easiest ways to use essential oils with babies are:

I. Diffusion

Diffusion involves diffusing essential oil in an oil burner or diffuser in order for it to disperse through the air and inhaled. For babies, simply add a drop of essential oil to 2 teaspoons of water and then add it to diffuser.

ii. Massage

To massage, create massage/body oil for your baby by combining essential oil with a carrier oil. Massage on the body so it penetrates the skin.

iii. Inhalation

Inhalation can be done with an inhaler, aroma lamp or with some cotton pads. If you use an inhaler, add 10 drops but only 2 drops with the cotton pads. Once the child inhales the oil from these, the therapeutic effects addresses the ailments which is usually a runny nose and congestion.

iv. Bath

For a calming effect and great scent, use the essential oils for the bath of children. Always dilute them in a carrier oil or in another carrier material. There is a big difference in diluting the oils for an adult and for a child. Children are more sensitive, so if you use 6 drops of essential oil to 20 ml of carrier oil for an adult, do not use more than 2-3 drops for a child.

Certain oils have repellent effects. They are effective against insect bites and in certain combinations, can keep nasty insects away from your child. You may also spray an essential oil combination or diffuse it, depending on their purpose.

Essential Oils That Are Good For Children

The correct usage of essential oil depends on the age of the baby. However, it is advisable to avoid using essential oils for babies under 3 months. This is because of their very tender skin which is also prone to allergic reactions.

For Babies 3Months And Above

Use 1-2 drops of essential oil/1ounce of carrier oil. The allowed essential oils include:

Chamomile (Roman and German)
Lavender
Yarrow (Blue)
Dill

For Babies Age 6 Months And Above

Increase the dose to 3-5 drops of essential oil/ 1ounce of carrier oil. The allowed essential oils Include:

Sweet Orange
Tangerine
Mandarin
Sandalwood
Tea tree
Bergamot
Citronella
Geranium
Grapefruit
Neroli
Palma Rosa
Pine
Cinnamon leaf – use very small amounts (1-2 drops). It can cause skin irritation if it is not diluted properly
Cinnamon bark – only use for diffusion. It is not safe to apply on the skin as it may cause severe irritation

Be careful with Citrus essential oils as they are photo toxic. What this means is they can cause severe reactions if the skin is exposed to sunlight. Do not use this kind of essential oils when preparing a sunscreen lotion, for example. Add lavender oil instead. There are a few citrus essential oils that are not photo toxic: Mandarin, Sweet Orange, Tangerine, Lemon or Lime obtained through steam distillation process.

For Children 2 Years And Above

Increase the dose to 20 drops of essential oil/1ounce of carrier oil. Choose from the list below:

Lime
Lemongrass
Frankincense
Basil, Lemon
Basil, Sweet
Melissa/Lemon Balm
Tea Tree, Lemon
Ylang Ylang
Sweet Marjoram
Garlic
Clary Sage
Thyme
Verbena, Lemon
Ginger
Oregano
Patchouli
Juniper Berry

For Children 6 Years And Above

Here, the list gets bigger and the dose too: 30 drops of essential oil/ounce of carrier oil. Essential oils to be used:

Nutmeg
Cardamom
Laurel Leaf/Bay Laurel
Niaouli
Peppermint
Cajuput
Anise, Star
Sage, Greek/White
Anise/Aniseed
Cornmint

Children 10 Years And Above

Here, all the essential oils are safe for diffusion or topical use. However, be careful with the oils you haven't used before. Introduce one at a time and test it before if it is applied on the skin.

Proper care should be taken when using essential oils that contain menthol and cineole. These two compounds may cause a reflex that slows down the breathing which, in some cases, can be dangerous.

There are 3 essential oils with these constituents:

Eucalyptus
Rosemary
Peppermint (at 6+ years, peppermint is safe for children's usage)

REMEDIES FOR COMMON AILMENTS

General Guidelines For Dilution

Babies 3+ months – 1-2 drops/1ounce of carrier oil (almond, grape seed, coconut oil)

Babies 6+ months – 3-5 drops/1ounce of carrier oil
Children 2+ years – 20 drops/1ounce of carrier oil

Children 6+ years old – 30 drops/1ounce of carrier oil

Fever
For babies

Ingredients

1-2 drops Lavender essential oil

1 oz carrier oil

Directions

Combine and massage child's feet, back, neck and behind the ears.

Sunburn
For young children

5 drops lavender

1 tsp aloe Vera

Directions

Dilute oil and apply over sunburned area.

Colds and Runny Nose
For young children

Ingredients

1 drop Lavender, Tea Tree, Thyme or Niaouli essential oil

1 oz carrier oil

Directions

Dilute and use for massaging baby's chest or back.

Flu
For young children

Ingredients

1 drop Cypress, lemon or Melaleuca

1 Tbsp. bath gel base

Directions

Dilute in a bath or diffuse

Diaper Rash
For babies

Ingredients

1-2 drops Lavender essential oil
1 oz carrier oil

Directions

Dilute & apply to the irritated area

Or

Ingredients

1 drop of Lavender essential oil

1 drop of Roman Chamomile essential oil

1 drop whole milk

Directions

Add to baby's bath water.

Before bathing baby, swish around

Do not let the oils get into your baby's eyes.

Common Cold Blend
For young children

Ingredients

2 drops Melaleuca (Tea Tree)

1 drop rose otto

1 drop lemon

2 Tbsp. vegetable oil

Directions

Combine and massage lightly on neck and chest.

Bruises
For young children

Ingredients

1 drop Lavender

1 drop Geranium

1 oz or 2 tbsp carrier oil

Directions

Dilute and apply to the bruise.

Minor Burns
For young children

Directions

1. Cool the skin for 10 minutes by immersing the burned skin in water.

2. If the skin isn't broken, apply 2 drops lavender essential oil directly on the burned area.

3. If the skin is broken, apply 2 drops of lavender around the burned area. Afterwards, put 5 drops of diluted lavender oil on a cold, dry cloth and then hold it over the area of the burn.

Colic Blend
For young children

Ingredients

1 drop of Roman Chamomile essential oil

1 drop Geranium

1 drop Lavender

2 tablespoons of almond oil

Directions

Blend and massage gently to the abdomen of the baby.

Cradle Cap
For babies

Ingredients

1 drop lemon

1 drop geranium

2 tbsp almond oil

Directions

Mix oils together and apply a small quantity on the head.

Crying
To soothe crying babies

Ingredients

1-2 drops Lavender or Roman Chamomile

Directions

Place on hand or tissue and offer the baby to smell.

Chicken Pox
For young children

Ingredients

10 drops lavender

10 drops Roman Chamomile

4 oz calamine lotion

Directions

1. Dilute oils in calamine lotion.

2. Mix well and apply over body two times daily

Cuts And Scrapes
For young children

Ingredients

5 drops lavender

5 drops Malaleuca

1 drop Lavender

Directions

1. Dilute oils in a small bowl of warm water.

2. Use the diluted water to clean the cut.

3. Apply 1 drop lavender essential oil to band- aid

4. Use it to cover the wound.

Coughs
For babies

Ingredients

1 drop of Lavender

1 tbsp carrier oil

Directions

Combine and rub a small quantity on baby's chest and back.

Diarrhea
For babies

Ingredients

1 drop Roman Chamomile

1 Tbsp carrier oil

Directions

1. Mix together and apply 2-3 drops of this mixture on the tummy.

2. Massage clockwise following the colon's natural movement.

Hiccoughs
For babies

Diffuse diluted Mandarin essential oil

Jaundice
For babies

Ingredients

1 drop Geranium

1 Tbsp carrier oil

Directions

Mix and apply over the liver area and to the bottoms of feet.

Earache
For young children

Ingredients

1-2 drops lavender

1-2 drops malaleuca

Directions

1. Dilute these oils and apply on a cotton pad.

2. Place the pad on the surface of the ear.

3. Place piece of tape across the ear to hold the cotton in place.

4. Send Child to bed.

Insect Bites
For babies & young children

Ingredients

1-2 drop lavender oil

2 tbsp or (1 oz) fractionated coconut oil

Directions

Dilute and dot each bite.

Constipation
For young children

Ingredients

1- 2 drops orange, mandarin or ginger essential oil

2tbs fractionated coconut oil

Directions

Dilute and massage a little on the feet.

Teething
For babies

Ingredients

1 drop lavender or Roman Chamomile

1 Tbsp carrier oil

Directions

Mix and use a little to massage gently along the jaw line.

Teeth grinding

Rub diluted Lavender essential oil on feet

Tummy Ache
For babies

Ingredients

1 drop Roman Chamomile

1 drop Sweet Orange

2 tbsp carrier oil

Directions

1. Mix and add 1 tsp of this mixture to warm bath water.

2. Before bathing baby, swish around and do not let the oils get into your baby's eyes.

Rashes
For young children

Ingredients

1 drop Lavender

1 drop Roman Chamomile

1 teaspoon fractionated oil

Directions

Combine and apply to location

Sleeping

Use this remedy on alternative nights until your baby learns to sleep all through the night.

Ingredients

1 drop chamomile Roman

1 drop geranium oil

1 bowl boiling water

Directions

1. Put your baby to bed and then place on the floor beneath the cot (crib) the bowl of boiling water.

2 Add the oils to it.

3. Leave the door ajar so the aroma molecules will be contained in the baby's room.

MASSAGE OILS AND LOTIONS

Homemade Baby Oil
Make your own baby oil to keep your baby happy and healthy

Suitable for babies 3 months + old

Ingredients

4 oz organic sweet almond oil
4 oz. organic olive oil

10 drops of Roman Chamomile essential oil

Directions

Combine the carrier oils and the Chamomile essential oil and mix well.

Baby Balm
Use this natural balm for eczema and other skin problems. It has an incredible scent too!

Suitable for children 6 months + old

Ingredients

¼ cup cocoa butter

¼ cup Shea butter

1 Tablespoon castor oil

2 Tablespoons olive oil

10 drops Sweet Orange Essential Oil

10 drops Sandalwood Essential Oil

Directions

1. Melt all the ingredients in a jar over a pan half full with water or a double boiler.

2. Let cool a little bit and add the essential oils.

3. Store in a container.

4. Massage the affected area with a small amount of baby balm.

Diaper Cream
Avoid using conventional diaper creams that contain chemical ingredients. Do it yourself!

This remedy is suitable for babies 6 months + old.

Ingredients

1/4 cup coconut oil

1/4 cup Shea butter

2 Tablespoons of Fermented Cod Liver Oil

1 Tablespoon beeswax pastilles

2 tablespoons of zinc oxide powder

1 tablespoon of bentonite clay

5 drops Chamomile essential oil

Directions

1. Combine Shea butter, beeswax and coconut oil and melt them in a double boiler.

2. Next, let it cool for 1 minute and then add the other ingredients.

3. Mix well and distribute the zinc oxide through the mixture.

4. Place it into the store container and stir a few more times until it's cool.

5. Keep in a dark place for 3 months.

Soft Baby Oil
Avoid the petroleum based baby oils and try this vitamin rich homemade oil

Suitable for babies 6 months + old

Ingredients

1 cup olive oil/apricot kernel oil

2 tablespoons calendula flowers

2 tablespoons chamomile flowers

10 drops Roman Chamomile essential oil

Directions

1. Place the herbs in a jar and cover them with the oil. Put a lid over the jar.

2. Store in a dark place for 6-8 weeks and shake every day.

3. Remove the flowers and add the essential oil

4. Use as regular baby oil.

Homemade Lotion for Babies

Your baby will love this ultra-moisturizing lotion.

Ingredients

¼ cup coconut oil

½ cup almond or olive oil

¼ cup beeswax

1 teaspoon Vitamin E oil

5 drops Lavender essential oil

5 drops Roman Chamomile essential oil

Directions

1. Melt the coconut oil, beeswax and almond/olive oil in a double boiler or a jar placed over a sauce pan half filled with hot water.

2. Once they melt, add the Vitamin E oil and the essential oils.

3. Store in a container.

Nourishing Baby Lotion

Protect your baby's skin with this smooth lotion

Suitable for babies 3 months + old

Ingredients

3 tablespoons cocoa butter

4 tablespoons apricot oil

1 tablespoon beeswax

1/2 cup filtered water

1 tablespoon dried lavender

5 drops Roman Chamomile essential oil

Directions

1. Combine the lavender and water and bring to a boil
2. Strain the tea and place it to a blender
3. Melt the cocoa butter and the beeswax.
4. To the melted mixture, add the apricot oil.
5. Place the oil mixture in the blender too.
6. Mix until it emulsifies.
7. Store in a jar and let it cool.

Rich Baby Oil
The blend of natural oils will nourish your baby's skin

Suitable for babies 3 months + old

Ingredients

2 oz apricot kernel oil

2 oz sweet almond oil

2 oz grape seed oil

1 tbsp Shea butter

1 tbsp cocoa butter

1 tbsp coconut butter

Few drops vitamin E oil

2 drops Lavender essential oil

Directions

1. Combine all the ingredients, except for the Vitamin E oil and the essential oil, and melt them into a double boiler.

2. Let cool for a few minutes, and then add the Vitamin E and Lavender essential oil. Store them in spray bottles.

Homemade Diaper Balm

Keep your baby happy with this soothing natural balm

Suitable for babies 3 months + old

Ingredients

1 oz cocoa butter

1 oz beeswax

3 oz Coconut oil

2 oz avocado oil

1 teaspoon Vitamin E oil

5 drops Lavender essential oil

5 drops Roman Chamomile essential oil

Directions

1. Combine the Cocoa butter, beeswax, coconut oil and avocado oil and place them in a double boiler or a jar over a saucepan half full with water.

2. Heat the ingredients until they melt, stirring a few times.

3. Let cool a little bit. Add the Vitamin E oil and the essential oils.

4. Store in a container.

Baby Smooth Balm

This balm can heal cuts, burns, rashes, scrapes, chapped lips.

Suitable for babies 6 months + old

Ingredients

½ cup of extra virgin olive oil

¼ cup dried calendula petals

1/8 cup of grated beeswax

8 drops of Lavender essential oil

Directions

1. Place the calendula petals and olive oil in a small slow cooker. Set the temperature on low for 3 hours.

2. Strain the oil very slowly. Mix the oil with the beeswax in a small skillet and let it heat until the beeswax melt.

3. After it cools for a few minutes, add the essential oil. Store in a dry container.

HYGIENE AND BATH

Homemade Shampoo & Body Wash
Suitable for babies 3 months + old if using only Lavender essential oil and for babies 6+ months old if using both essential oils

Ingredients

4 oz filtered water
1 oz liquid castile soap, unscented
3 drops Sweet Orange essential oil
3 drops Lavender essential oil

Directions

Mix all the ingredients in a container.

Lavender Baby Shampoo
This homemade shampoo is distinguished through its delicate lavender smell

Suitable for babies 6 months + old

Ingredients

1 cup castile soap

4 cups distilled water

1/4 cup aloe Vera gel

2 tablespoons coconut oil

3 teaspoons guar gum

1.5 teaspoon Neo Defend

2 teaspoons citric acid

30 drops Lavender essential oil

Directions

1. Put all the ingredients, except the castile soap, in a blender and mix for about 40 sec

2. Add the castile soap

3. Place the shampoo into a container.

Baby Powder
Instead of using talc on your baby's skin, try this homemade recipe.

Suitable for babies 6 months + old

Ingredients

½ cup arrowroot powder

5 drops Roman Chamomile essential oil

Directions

Combine the ingredients and store in a container.

Chamomile Baby Shampoo
This homemade shampoo will fit perfectly to your baby's soft hair.

Suitable for babies 6 months + old

Ingredients

6 oz castile soap

1 teaspoon almond oil

10 drops Roman Chamomile essential oil

Directions

1. Mix well all the ingredients

2. Store in a clean container.

Teething Gel
Suitable for infants 2 years + old

1 drop Clove Essential Oil

1 tablespoon glycerine or vegetable oil

Directions

Combine in small bottle, shaking until thoroughly blended.

Milk Bath
Milk can be used as a nourishing bath additive for babies

Suitable for babies 3 months + old.

Ingredients

1/2 cup cornstarch

1 cup dried milk

2 to 3 drops Lavender or Chamomile essential oils

Directions

1. Mix all ingredients thoroughly.

2. Put a small amount of this mixture in the warm bath.

Homemade Baby Powder
Say no to diaper rash with this natural baby powder.

Suitable for babies 6 months + old

Ingredients

1/4 cup arrowroot powder

1/4 cup cornstarch

1 tbsp white clay

3 drops Sweet Orange essential oil

1 drop Geranium essential oil

2 drops Sandalwood essential oil

Directions

Mix the ingredients and store in a jar.

Homemade Baby Wipes
Use this all natural baby wipes for your baby's hygiene.

Suitable for babies 6 months +

Ingredients

1/8-1/4 cup Castile soap

2 cups lukewarm water

1/8-1/4 cup vegetable oil (almond, olive, apricot seeds, etc)

Roll of paper towels

1 plastic container that the roll will fit in

5 drops Chamomile essential oil

2 drops Tea Tree essential oil

Directions

1. Take the roll of paper towels and cut it in half, then remove the cardboard.

2. Mix all the ingredients in the container.

3. Put the paper roll in the container, cut side down.

4. Seal the container and turn it upside down.

5. Pull the wipes from the middle in order to use.

Baby Healing Wipes

These natural baby wipes have a comforting effect on your baby's skin

Suitable for babies 6 months + old

Ingredients

1/4 cup Aloe Vera gel

1 1/2 to 2 cups distilled water

2 teaspoon castile soap

1 tablespoon Calendula oil

2 to 3 drops Tea Tree oil

2 to 3 drops Lavender oil

Roll of paper towels

1 plastic container that the roll will fit in

Directions

1. Mix all the ingredients, apart from the essential oils

2. Let the mixture sit for a few minutes, then add the essential oils

3. Take the roll of paper towels and cut it in half, then remove the cardboard.

4. Place the mixture into the container.

5. Put the paper roll in the container, cut side down.

6. Seal the container and turn it upside down.

7. Pull the wipes from the middle in order to use.

Baby Bubble Bath
Let your baby enjoy his/her bath with natural bubbles.

Ingredients

3/4 cup water

1 cup baby shampoo or eco-friendly liquid soap

1/2 to1 teaspoon glycerin

2 drops Chamomile essential oil

2 drops Lavender essential oil

Directions

Mix all the ingredients and let them sit for a while before adding the essential oils.

SUNSCREEN LOTIONS

Homemade Sunscreen

Use a homemade lotion that protects and nourishes the skin of your baby.

Suitable for babies 6 months + old

Ingredients

¼ cup of Shea butter

¼ cup of coconut oil

2 tablespoons beeswax granules

1/8 cup almond oil

1-2 tablespoons of zinc oxide

10 drops Lavender essential oil

Directions

1. Place the coconut oil, Shea butter, beeswax and almond oil in a jar.

2. Heat some water in a saucepan and put the jar inside or use a double boiler. Wait for all the ingredients to melt.

3. Next, mix in the zinc oxide and refrigerate for 10 minutes. (Always use a mask when dealing with zinc oxide. Be sure to distribute it all throughout the mixture).

4. Take it out, add the Lavender essential oil and blend all the ingredients using a hand mixer.

5. Put the sunscreen in a container and use it within 6 months. Store in a dark place.

Natural Homemade Sunscreen

Protect your baby from skin irritation with this remedy

Suitable for children 6 months + old

Ingredients

1 oz coconut oil

0.8 oz shea butter
0.1 oz Vitamin E oil

0.1 oz jojoba, sesame, or sunflower oil

1 tablespoon zinc oxide powder

10 drops Lavender/Sandalwood essential oil

Directions

1. Use a double boiler to melt the following ingredients: Shea butter, coconut oil and jojoba/sunflower/sesame oil.

2. Remove the oily mixture and let it cool.

3. Using a mask, add the vitamin E oil, essential oils and the zinc oxide and evenly distribute.

4. Move the sunscreen into a container and store in a dark place.

INSECT REPELLENTS FOR CHILDREN

Homemade Insect Repellent

Did you know that all store-bought repellents contain DEET which may not be 100% safe for your children? Protect your kids today! Make your own repellent.

Suitable for children 2 years +

Ingredients

15 drops citronella essential oil
10 drops lemongrass essential oil

10 drops lemon essential oil

5 drops cedar essential oil

1 oz witch hazel

1 oz grape seed oil

Directions

1. Mix all the ingredients in a spray bottle

2. Shake thoroughly before applying on skin.

Water Based Bug Spray

It and protects your child from the nasty insects.

Suitable for children 2 years + old

Ingredients

2 oz water

2 oz witch hazel/vodka/apple cider vinegar

¼ teaspoon castile soap

10 drops citronella essential oil

10 drops lemongrass essential oil

10 drops tea tree oil

5 drops cedar essential oil

5 drops lemon essential oil

Directions

1. Mix the essential oils with the witch hazel/vodka/apple cider vinegar.

2. Add the castile soap and let it still for a few minutes.

3. Shake well the mixture.

4. Add the water.

5. Place the liquid into a spray bottle.

6. Shake before use

Oil Based Bug Spray
Suitable for children 2 years + old

Ingredients

2 oz jojoba or olive oil

10 drops citronella essential oil

10 drops lemongrass essential oil

10 drops tea tree oil

5 drops cedar essential oil

5 drops lemon essential oil

Directions

Mix all the ingredients and store in spray bottle.

Patchouli Bug Spray
The blend of essential oils smells great and will keep insects away.

Suitable for children 2 years + old

Ingredients

4 oz witch hazel/vodka/apple cider vinegar

15 drops patchouli essential oil

10 drops geranium essential oil

15 drops cedarwood atlas or cedarwood Virginia essential oil

Directions

1. Mix the essential oils to the witch hazel/vodka/apple cider vinegar and let it sit for a while.

2. After that mix well and add the water.

3. Store it in a spray bottle.

4. Shake well before use.

Wonder Bug Spray
Suitable for children 2 years + old

Ingredients

2 oz jojoba or olive oil

13 drops geranium bourbon essential oil

13 drops patchouli essential oil

13 drops cedarwood atlas or cedarwood Virginia essential oil

Directions

Mix all the ingredients and store in spray bottle.

Citronella Spray
Citronella essential oil with its strong repellent effect works excellently.

Suitable for children 2 years + old

Ingredients

2 oz water

2 oz witch hazel/vodka/apple cider vinegar

15 drops cedarwood atlas or cedarwood Virginia essential oil

15 drops citronella essential oil

10 drops geranium essential oil

Directions

1. Mix the essential oils to the witch hazel/vodka/apple cider vinegar and let it sit for a while.

2. After that mix well and add the water.

3. Store it in a spray bottle.

4. Shake well before use.

Soothing Insect Spray
Use only natural ingredients for protecting your child's skin.

Suitable for children 2 years + old

Ingredients

2 oz jojoba/olive oil

15 drops cedarwood atlas or cedarwood Virginia essential oil

15 drops citronella essential oil

10 drops geranium essential oil

Directions

Mix all the ingredients and store in a spray bottle.

Itchy Relief Repellent

Get rid of all annoying itches with this natural repellent.

Suitable for children 2 years + old

Ingredients

2 oz jojoba/coconut oil

10 drops neem oil

10 drops Lavender essential oil

10 drops Lemon essential oil

10 drops Thyme essential oil

10 drops Geranium essential oil

Directions

Mix all the ingredients and store in a bottle.

HOUSE CLEANING

Homemade Laundry Soap

Don't let all the harsh chemicals from conventional detergents touch the skin of your baby.

Suitable for babies 3 months + old

Ingredients

3 tablespoons washing soda

3 tablespoons borax

2 tablespoons organic dish soap

15 drops Lavender essential oil

4 cups boiling water

Directions

1. Mix together: borax, washing soda, dish soap and essential oils in a large container (one gallon)

2. Pour the boiling water and stir until well combined

3. Let this mixture cool.

4. Fill the container with cold water almost to the top

Homemade Liquid Laundry Soap

The soap nuts are the most harmless washing agent ever! They are just perfect for your baby's clothes.

Suitable for babies 6 months + old.

Ingredients

1 cup soap nuts

1/2 cup vinegar (natural preservative)

4 cups water

10 drops Sweet Orange essential oil

10 drops Tangerine essential oil

Directions

1. Place the soap nuts, vinegar and water into a large pot and mix them together.

2. Bring to a boil on medium-low temperature and let them simmer for 30 minutes. The lid must be on the pot.

3. Remove the lid and let boil for 30 minutes more. Stir from time to time.

4. Let the liquid cool and add the essential oils.

5. Sore into a clean container.

Perfect Stain Remover

We all know how babies' clothes can get very dirty. However, this natural stain remover will help.

Ingredients

1/4 cup liquid castile soap

1 1/2 cups water

1/4 cup liquid vegetable glycerin

5-10 drops of Lemon essential oil

Directions

1. Combine all the ingredients and mix well.

2. Store in a glass container (Lemon essential oil may have a harsh effect on plastic)

Boom Liquid Dishwasher

When you wash your child's dishes there can be detergent leftovers. It is best to use a natural dishwasher in order to protect your baby.

Ingredients

1/8 cup water

1/2 cup liquid castile soap

4 drops essential oil scent of choice

1 teaspoon vinegar

Directions

Combine all the ingredients and store into an old dishwasher container.

Homemade Toy Cleaner
A cheap way to keep your child's toys clean.

Ingredients

1 cup distilled white vinegar

1 cup water

3 drops Tea Tree essential oil

Directions

Mix all the ingredients and store in spray bottle.

Homemade Surface Cleaner
Keep your house clean for the safety of your children

Ingredients

2 tablespoons white vinegar

1 1/2 cups of warm water in a measuring cup

1 teaspoon liquid castile soap

2 teaspoons rubbing alcohol

8-10 drops of Tea Tree essential oil (for its antibacterial effect)

1 citrus peel

Directions

1. Combine all the ingredients and mix well.

2. Store in a spray bottle.

Safe Surface Cleaner
Ingredients

8 drops Mandarin essential oil

1 cup water

Directions

Combine to a spray bottle.

Use to wipe down surfaces in baby's room.

Citrus Surface Cleaner
Ingredients

1 cup distilled vinegar

1 cup water

½ lemon, juiced

10 drops Sweet Orange essential oil

Directions

1. Mix all the ingredients.

2. Store in a spray bottle

BOOK 3

Essential Oils For Family Health

Simple Aromatherapy Recipes For Common Ailments

Coral Miller

INTRODUCTION

Essential oils are the potent and aromatic liquids extracted from the leaves, seeds, fruits, barks, flowers, roots or seeds of plants, herbs and shrubs. Essential oils are generally created through distillation, a process which separates the oil and water- based plant compounds by steaming.

Essential oils are highly concentrated oils with a strong aroma. Being highly concentrated, just one drop is sufficient to create powerful health benefits. What this means is that we are literally separating the most powerful healing compounds of a particular plant into one single oil. For example, to get a pound of lavender essential oil will require 150 pounds of lavender flowers! Do you see how highly concentrated essential oils are? So essentially (no pun meant), you will be getting 150 times the healing properties from lavender essential oils than you would get from using straight lavender.

The reason why these natural oils are in plants in the first place is to protect them (the plant) from insects and a harsh environment. So when you take essential oils, you will be harnessing the plant's healing and protective powers. Of a truth, essential oils are the most potent form of plant based medicine. So effective is their power to heal and cure diseases that a lot of people can now successfully avoid taking a plethora of medications or undergoing various surgeries simply by taking essential oils correctly.

Why Essential Oils Are So Powerful

Essential oils are made of tiny molecules that can penetrate your cells. Some compounds in certain essential oils can even cross the blood-brain barrier. Fatty oils from vegetables or nuts come from large molecules so they cannot penetrate your cells. As a result, they are not therapeutic in any way. Unlike essential oils, vegetable oils are not small enough to get into your system so they can only stay on your skin and may end up even clogging your pores.

Essential oils are transdermal. When placed anywhere on the body, they pass through the skin and straight into the circulatory system and cells. They are so powerful that they are often diluted with a carrier oil such as coconut or olive oil before they can be used. Since they can travel through the body and the air (via diffusion) at an incredibly rate, they have great health benefits.

Think about this: if you had peppermint leaves in your kitchen, you probably wouldn't be able to smell them from 12 feet away, could you? But if you are diffusing peppermint or cinnamon essential oils you will be able to smell them throughout your home!

The reason for this is the volatile compounds that are in essential oils moves through your olfactory system (your sense of smell) to your cells and into your blood stream within seconds. So if your child is ill, you can diffuse clove and frankincense essential oils in the air to aid quick recovery and to keep your entire family healthy.

Once these oil compounds are in your system, they can protect and heal your body in a variety of ways. This is what is known as aromatherapy: natural healing from essential oils. At this juncture, it will be safe to mention that medicinal tinctures and dried herbs can also heal. Ground ginger root and cinnamon have lots of health benefits as well. Eating healthy foods like fresh herbs and vegetables can also support healing. Nevertheless, in terms of compounds with the strongest concentrated healing properties, essential oils surpass them all.

Quality Of Essential Oils

Not all essential oils are created the same. In fact, most of them are potentially toxic and worthless to your health. There are four grades of essential oils:

1. Synthetic and Altered Oils are the lowest grade of oil. They are created in laboratory.

2. Natural and "Pure" Oils. They are the most commonly sold type of oils. They are usually over-processed so they lose their healing compounds.

3. Wellness Grade Essential Oils; these are steam distilled with healing compounds. The only setback is that they may have been sprayed with pesticides.

4. Certified Therapeutic Grade Essential Oils; these are the highest grade of essential oils with maximum healing properties.

Only the highest quality essential oils can promote healing. To create true quality essential oils, the quality of plants and the quality of processing are important. High quality plants must be planted in nutrient dense organic soil and must be harvested when their healing compounds are most available.

The next step should is to extract the oils using steam distillation or cold pressed and not chemicals. Finally, bottle the oils in dark glass containers to protect from sunlight and oxidation. Ensure you buy therapeutic grade and organic oils at all times when purchasing essential oils.

How To Use Essential Oils

There are 3 main ways essential oils can be used: topical, inhalation and internal.

Topical Use

This involves applying essential oils on the skin, either directly or directly. A few oils can be applied directly on the skin e.g. lavender but most oils must be mixed with a carrier oil before usage. Some of the best carrier oils include jojoba oil, coconut oil, olive oil, almond oil and pomegranate seed oil.

Key points of application on the body are:

- Behind ears
- Abdomen
- Neck
- Temples
- Soles and tops of feet
- Along spine
- Upper back

Other topical ways to use oils include:

Baths: essential oils can be used as aromatherapy baths.. This could help improve circulation, relax the body, relieve sore muscles, open airways, improve sleep and soothe the skin. It is best to mix the oils with bath salts, milk or sesame oil for quick dispersion. Failure to do this will cause the oils to float on water and even stick to your skin directly. Use soothing oils like lavender and eucalyptus. Additionally, the bath could either be a full body bath or foot bath.

Compresses: compresses work well for infections, bruises, aches and pains. Simply add your preferred essential oil to bowl of either hot or cold water. (It could be diluted with carrier, depending on the treatment). Dip a clean cloth in the water, wring it out and place on the affected area. Peppermint works real well for muscle aches and lavender is just great for infections.

Salves: to make salves, mix coconut oil, vitamin E oil, beeswax and essential oils. Store in a metal or glass container and rub as needed. Salves are very effective for cuts, scrapes, bruises or sore muscle.

Massage: Aromatherapy massage is another effective topical application. Make sure that you always dilute with suitable carrier oil.

Inhalation

Diffusion is another excellent way to use essential oil. You can either use diffusers or inhale the oil directly in hot water. Inhalations are highly effective for headaches, respiratory and sinus problems. Only ensure that you inhale for 2- 3 minutes at a stretch. Inhaling essential oils for too long can cause nausea, dizziness and headaches.

Internal Use

Internal use of essential oils can only be effective if pure therapeutic grade oils are used. Dosage and dilution is also dependent on the individual's age, size and health. However, it is best to consult your physician or nutritionist before ingesting any essential oil.

Ways by which essential oils can be taken internally include:

- Putting a few drops in an empty capsule and swallowing with water
- Putting 1-3 drops of oil to 1 teaspoon of coconut oil then consume.
- Adding 1-3 drops of oil to a glass of coconut milk, water or almond milk.
- Adding 1-3 drops of oil to 1 teaspoon of raw honey.

Top Essential Oils For Healing

Stock these six essential oils in your medicine cabinet and keep your family healthy all year long.

Tea Tree

Also called Melaleuca, tea tree is a powerful antifungal, antibacterial and antiseptic oil. It can be used topically to treat all sorts of skin problems. You only need a few drops diluted with a carrier oil and your cuts, scrapes, acne blemishes, insect bites, ringworm, warts, fungal infections, athletic foot and even dandruff will be eliminated. It can also help to boost the immune system. In some cases, it can even be used undiluted. It is found in a lot of skin care products.

Uses

- Mix 5 drops with 1 tablespoon of raw honey and use mixture as acne free -face wash.
- Apply to ringworm, Candida, athlete's foot or other fungal infections.
- Put directly on mosquito, spider or bug bites to detox poison.
- Add 5 drops to your favorite shampoo to reduce dandruff and to improve scalp health.
- Kick a cold or flu by gargling tea tree oil and water.
- Mix 2 teaspoon of melaleuca and water in a spray bottle for an all-purpose cleaner.
- Diffuse in the air to purify it of mold and allergens.

Lavender

One of the most versatile oils, lavender has antiviral and antibacterial properties and it is effective on cuts, bruises and general skin care. It doesn't always require a carrier oil and can be applied directly to the affected area. It is relaxing and uplifting, helping to balance hormones in women and generally reducing the stress hormones in the body.

Uses

- To relax the body and improve sleep, rub on neck in the evenings.
- To restore the body after a long day, add a few drops to your bath along with some Epsom salts.
- Put on your kids' cuts, bruises, scrapes, burns, rashes, and wounds.
- Diffuse in the air improve mood and relax.
- Use topically on neck to lower cholesterol& blood pressure or take as supplement.

Peppermint:

Peppermint is cooling, it stimulates the mind and increases mental alertness. For an instant cooling effect, simply dilute with a carrier and rub on your chest, back and neck. Peppermint oil wards off nausea, morning or motion sickness.

It reduces headaches and migraines to a large extent when applied to the temple. It has antimicrobial properties as well so also helps to freshen bad breath and treat digestive issues such as flatulence, indigestion and slow digestion.

Uses

- Mix with coconut oil or carrier oil of choice and rub topically on sore muscles.
- Diffuse it in air to improve energy and focus.
- To improve breathing and fight infections, rub on bottom of feet& chest
- Mix with baking soda and coconut oil for homemade toothpaste.
- Freshen breath, put 1 drop in clean water.
- To improve digestion & reduce nausea, take 1 drop in water.

Lemon

Lemon oil is effective in its ability to detox every part of the body. With its uplifting properties, it is also good for improved focus, concentration and to rejuvenate energy. It helps treat wounds and infections and acts as a powerful bug repellent.

Uses

- To freshen breath, put 1-2 drops in water.
- To promote cleansing & metabolism, take 1 drop as supplement three times daily.
- To uplift mood, diffuse to clean air and enjoy a nice citrus scent.
- Improve home smell by diffusing in the air.
- Rub on hands in instead of hand sanitizer for its antimicrobial benefits.
- Mix with baking soda as all- natural teeth whitener.
- Mix with olive oil and use as natural cleaning product.

Frankincense

A very powerful essential oil, frankincense was valued above gold in ancient times due its ability to treat all sorts of illnesses. Recent research has shown that it is even more effective than chemotherapy in shrinking tumors and killing cancer cells. It helps to reduce inflammation and improve immune function. It also fights infections, heals acne, sunspot and skin scarring.

Uses

- To improve immunity, rub topically on neck, chest, behind ears and to bottoms of feet.
- Apply to minor cuts for healing and pain relief.
- To reduce scars, age spots and stretch marks, dilute oil and apply once or twice a day.
- Use after a trauma to calm yourself.

- Rub topically on areas of joint pain
- To relieve stress and headaches, apply to temples with lavender.
- Add to baths for extra relaxation.
- Diffuse in air to reduce seasonal allergies

Eucalyptus

This is a powerful antiviral, antibacterial and antispasmodic oil that works on coughs, colds and allergies that affect breathing. To clear your nasal passages and lungs, just add a few drops to a vaporizer or to bowl of steaming water and inhale. It stimulates the immune system and loosens congested chest. Prevent a full cold also by using regularly during cold season.

COLDS & COUGHS

Cough Mixture

2 drops Eucalyptus oil

2 drops Lemon oil

3 tablespoons honey

What To Do

1. Mix the oil and honey together.

2. Use 1 teaspoon of this mixture in half a glass of warm water.

3. Sip slowly.

Vapor Rub
For chest congestion

5 drops peppermint oil

12 drops eucalyptus oil

1 ounce olive oil

5 drops thyme oil

What To Do

1. Add all ingredients to a glass bottle, shaking to mix well.

2. Massage gently into throat and chest.

3. Use daily and always before bed time.

Power Chest Rub

For Coughs & Chest Congestion

Ingredients

2 tbsp virgin coconut oil or Shea butter

7 drops Peppermint essential oil

1/3 cup jojoba or olive oil

2 drops Cedarwood essential oil

15 drops Eucalyptus essential oil

1 drop Thyme essential oil

What To Do

1. Pour 1 inch water (2.5cm) in a medium-sized pot bottom and heat on low until it simmers.

2. Place the coconut oil or Shea butter in Pyrex or measuring cup. Place the Pyrex in the water and warm gently on low heat until the butter melts.

3. Remove from the heat, add the olive or jojoba oil and stir.

4. Pour the oil mixture into a PET or dark glass jar. Add the essential oils.

5. Wait for 24-36 hours before using. Store bottle in a cool and dark place.

Caution: Do not use Thyme essential oil if you have sensitive skin because it may cause irritation. This is the reason it's at a low concentration. Also, avoid eucalyptus if you have epilepsy or high blood pressure.

Colds

The symptoms of a cold include a sore throat, stuffed-up, runny nose, dry cough and sneezing. Flu is much more serious than a cold, but tends to display similar symptoms.

2 drops lavender

2 drops eucalyptus

2 drops rosemary

2 teaspoons milk or cream

What To Do

1. Add oils to cream or milk.

2. Pour into a warm bath and enjoy.

Colds & Flu Home Spray

1 drop Pine essential oil

1 drop Cinnamon essential oil

1 drop Eucalyptus essential oil

1 drop Cloves essential oil

1 drop Niaouli essential oil

500 ml water

1. Mix the oils in the water and place in a spray can.

2. Shake well to mix the oils well and spray the home.

Anti-Flu Bath

Flu is a severe form of cold. It causes body aches, high fever, chills, exhaustion and muscle sores. Flu viruses are more infectious, more harmful and often stronger than those of colds. They are highly contagious as well.

4 drops Tea tree oil

1 drop of Lemon oil

3 drops Lavender oil

What To Do

Add these oils to a warm bath.

After bath, also massage by combining these oils:

Anti- Flu Massage
3 drops Tea tree oil

2 drops Eucalyptus oil

10 ml Evening primrose oil

Cold Sores Quick Fix

Cold sores are small painful blisters around the lips. They are caused by an outbreak of herpes simplex virus that shows up when stress levels are high. They are called cold sores because the sores usually accompany colds.

1. Use 2 drops Tea tree oil neat or Calendula oil, Chamomile oil or Geranium essential oil diluted in carrier oil.

2. Apply directly onto sore to relieve the pain and swelling.

Cold Sores Blend

4 drops Geranium Essential Oil

2 drops Chamomile Essential Oils

3 drops Tea Tree Essential Oils

1 drop Lavender Essential Oils

10 ml Aloe Vera Gel

What To Do

1. To a 10 ml glass jar, add the Aloe Vera Gel to fill 2/3 of jar.

2. Add the essential oils and mix with spoon. Now fill jar and remix.

3. Apply as prevention when the tingling feeling start or apply direct onto sore to encourage healing.

Kid's Cold Cure

10 drops Lavender

10 drops Eucalyptus

10 drops Tea Tree

What To Do

1. Combine all oils. Put 3 drops of mixture in a diffuser at bedtime.

2. For heavy congestion, put 2 drops of the mixture on cotton piece and tuck it inside the child's pillowcase at night.

3. Put 2 to 5 drops in a bath. The steam will help to clear the nasal passages and help your child to rest.

Nasal Inhaler
For Chest Congestion

5 drops of eucalyptus essential oil

1/4 teaspoon of coarse salt

What To Do

1. Put the salt in a small glass vial. Add the essential oil.

2. Open the vial and inhale deeply as needed all through the day.

Ease Sinus Congestion
2 drops Tea Tree

2 drops Eucalyptus

2 drops Peppermint

What To Do

1. Add oils to steaming pot of water.

2. Cover the pot and head immediately with a towel.

3. Inhale for 3 minutes, keeping eyes closed.

Night-Time Colds & Flu Combater
2 drops Lavender

2 drops Tea Tree

What To Do

1. Add oils to a steaming bowl of water.

2. Let the steam diffuses into the room.

3. Alternatively, add oils to a tea candle diffuser.

SKIN INJURIES & BOO-BOOS

Blisters

Blisters are painful swelling on the skin. It is caused by fluid accumulation underneath the skin. Once the blister bursts, the exposed tissue beneath could become infected. Injury, burning, an insect sting, scalding or chafing could result in blisters.

What To Do

1. Simply apply a drop of tea tree oil or lavender onto the blister.

2. Carefully but thoroughly pat in.

Grazes

Children will always run around and may hurt themselves. Protect them from infection when grazes occur.

What To Do

1. Take out the splinter.

2. Bath all dirt thoroughly by using 10 drops lavender, tea tree, lemon or Eucalyptus in a bowl of warm water.

3. Let the damaged skin remain open in the fresh air. If there is danger of re-infection, make sure you cover-up.

Emergency Burn Wash/Compress
5 drops lavender oil

1 pint water, about 50°F

What To Do

1. Add the oil to the water, stirring well to disperse the oil.

2. Soak a soft cloth in the water and then apply to the burn. Let it stay for 5-10 minutes. Repeat process twice.

3. Alternatively, immerse the burned area directly in the water for 5 minutes.

Bruise
A bruise is a skin discoloration that occurs when blood leaks from damaged blood vessels into the surrounding tissues under the skin. Bruises usually heal naturally but you could use the remedy below for an extra boost.

5 drops Calendula oil

2 drops Fennel oil

1 drop Cypress oil

10 ml Grape seed oil

What To Do

1. Dilute essential oils in carrier oil and massage the affected area.

Minor Burns
2 drops lavender

What To Do

1. Apply ice cold water immediately to the burn for 10 minutes.

2. Apply 2 drops neat lavender onto it.

Insect Bites
1. Remove the sting by applying a few drops of neat lavender oil to it

Insect Repellent Spray
2 ounces distilled water

1.5 ounces witch hazel or vodka

25 drops peppermint oil

30 drops citronella oil

15 drops tea tree oil

1 teaspoon of jojoba oil (optional but if you add this, add only 1 oz of witch hazel or vodka)

<u>What To Do</u>

1. Add the vodka or witch hazel to a 4 oz clean spray bottle filled with distilled or boiled water.

2. Add the essential oils and shake thoroughly. Spray onto clothing and/or exposed skin but avoid the eyes and mucous membranes.

3. Reapply as needed. Store it in a dark bottle and away from sunlight or heat. This makes 4 ounces

Antiseptic Cream
For cuts and wounds

20 drops Lavender Essential Oil

15 drops Tea Tree Essential Oil

15 drops Geranium Essential Oil

43 ml Base Cream

What To Do

1. Add the Base Cream to a fill 2/3 of 50 ml dark colored glass jar.

2. Add essential oils, mixing with a spoon. Fill jar

3. Use directly onto injury, cover with bandage for quicker healing.

Wounds
Wounds must be sterilized to prevent infection.

2 drops Tea Tree oil

5 drops Lavender oil

500 ml warm water

What To Do

1. Combine oils in water and bathe the wound area.

2. Cover up the wound by dropping 3 drops of Lavender oil on a piece of gauze and then placing it over the cut.

3. Renew two times daily. On the third day, expose the wound to air if possible.

Bleeding

Bleeding should always be taken seriously, regardless of what kind it is. An adult usually has about 5 liter of blood. Even the loss of 1 liter can be fatal.

<u>For a small open wound:</u>

1 drop Chamomile oil

1 drop Geranium oil

1 drop Lemon oil

1 drop Tea Tree oil

<u>What To Do</u>

1. Combine and apply as a compress.

Cuts Spray
To reduce the risk of infection

6 drops eucalyptus oil

12 drops tea tree oil

6 drops of lemon oil

2 oz distilled water

<u>What To Do</u>

1. Combine all the ingredients, shaking well before each use.

2. Dispense as needed from a spray bottle. Use on minor cuts, burns or abrasions to speed healing and prevent infection.

Boils

Boils are abscesses usually found at the buttocks or underarms. Fever and fatigue can be associated with boils as well.

Ingredients

2 drops Tea tree oil

2 drops Lavender oil

1 drop Juniper oil

200 ml hot water

What To Do

1. Dilute the essential oils in the hot water.

2. For severe inflammation, add 1 drop Chamomile oil.

3. Bathe the area two times daily.

4. Alternatively, apply undiluted tea tree or lavender oil to the area using a cotton bud.

Anti- Abscess Compress

An abscess is typically caused by bacteria and forms around a hair follicle. Generally, however, it is a pus- filled cavity where the skin becomes red and swollen and later develops into a throbbing elevated lump.

2 drops Tea Tree essential oil

2 drops Lavender essential oil

2 drops Chamomile essential oil

Combine and apply to the area of swelling twice daily.

HEADACHES

A headache is simply a pain in the head but the severity of the discomfort varies to a great extent. Headaches are symptomatic. The underlying cause could be stress, tension, fatigue, allergies or blocked sinuses. Others include drug overuse, adverse reaction to medication and seasonal changes.

Fast Fix Remedy
3 drops lavender essential oils

2 drops peppermint essential oils

What To Do

1. Add oils to fold-up tissue.

2. Inhale slowly and deeply in 3 long breaths.

3. Repeat three times.

Anti- Headache Blend
1 drop Peppermint oil

3 drops Lavender oil

3 drops Jojoba oil

1 drop Bergamot oil

What To Do

1. Mix oils and massage around the temples or into the base of the skull.

Tension/ Nervous Headache Mix
1 drop Clary sage oil

3 drops of Lavender oil

2 drops of Jojoba oil

1 drop Chamomile oil

<u>What To Do</u>

1. Mix oils and massage around the temples or into the base of the skull.

Headache Balm
1 tablespoon Beeswax, grated

1/4 cup Shea Butter

1/4 teaspoon (or 1 capsule) Vitamin E

1 tablespoon Grapeseed oil

8 drops Lavender essential oil

1 drop Chamomile essential oil

1 drop Jasmine essential oil

<u>What To Do</u>

1. Place the beeswax, Shea butter & grapeseed oil in a double boiler over a low heat until melted.

2. Remove from heat; add the essential oils and the vitamin E. Pour into a dark glass jar and store in a cool, dark place.

3. Rub onto back of your neck and your temples to ease pain and soothe tension.

STOMACH RELIEF

Diarrhea

Diarrhea is the frequent and excessive discharge of the bowel movement, signaling that something is not right with the system. It could be caused by eating spicy foods, undigested vegetables, unripe fruits, excessive food consumption, eating too fast and drinking unclean water.

<u>A massage oil to help ease diarrhea</u>

2 drops Lavender essential oil

2 drops Peppermint essential oil

2 drops Eucalyptus essential oil

2 drops Chamomile essential oil

2 drops Geranium essential oil

10 ml vegetable carrier oil

Combine and rub over the abdomen area.

Hiccups

Hiccups are not meant to last for a long time otherwise they can be very painful.

<u>What To Do</u>

1. Place 1 drop Chamomile essential oil in a brown paper bag.

2. Hold the bag over your nose and mouth.

3. Breathe in slowly and deeply through your nose.

Stomach Massage
For indigestion

2 drops Cinnamon

4 drops Peppermint

6 drops Mandarin

2 tablespoons carrier oil

<u>What To Do</u>

1. Dilute essential oils with the carrier oil.

2. Massage onto stomach.

Nausea Instant Remedy
The underlying cause of nausea can be physiological, psychological or both. Reasons such as disgusting smells, hangovers, bad digestion, food poisoning, motion sickness, early pregnancy and tonsillitis could contribute to nausea.

1 drop of Lavender essential oil

1 drop Peppermint essential oil

1 drop Basil essential oil

2 teaspoons (10ml) carrier oil of choice

<u>What To Do</u>

1. Combine all the oils. Massage over your abdomen very gently.

2. Cup your hands over your mouth & nose and then inhale a few times slowly. Wash your hands.

Motion Sickness

1. Add 2 drops lavender or bergamot essential oil to a handkerchief and sniff.

2. Get enough fresh air.

Heartburn

Heartburn is an uncomfortable burning pain in the lower chest. It often occurs after a meal when the stomach acids flows back into the esophagus' lower end.

2 drops Eucalyptus oil

2 drops Fennel oil

1 drop Peppermint oil

1 teaspoon (5ml) Grape seed oil

What To Do

1. Dilute the essential oils in the carrier oil

2. Rub the upper abdominal area with this mixture.

Bladder Infection Oil

6 drops tea tree oil

8 drops juniper berry or cypress oil

2 drops fennel oil

6 drops bergamot oil

2 ounces vegetable oil

What To Do

1. Combine all ingredients. Massage once a day over the bladder area.

2. For prevention, add 1 tablespoon of this mixture to your bath.

Bladder Infection Sitz Bath
5 drops lavender oil

5 drops rosemary oil

<u>What To Do</u>

1. Add the essential oils to hot bath

2. Sit for 5-10 minutes in a tub with the hot water up to the waist.

3. Next, switch to a tub of cold water for at 1-2 minute. Do 2-5 rounds.

4. Do this treatment daily or at least two times a week.

PAINS

For Rheumatism & Arthritis

3 drops Chamomile

3 drops Lavender

3 drops Yarrow

3 drops Eucalyptus

8 ounces sweet-almond oil

Add the essential oils to almond oil

Massage into affected areas.

Massage Oil For Abdominal Pain

Abdominal pain may be caused by eating too fast, digestive problems or menstruation.

1 drop of Chamomile oil

1 drop Peppermint oil

1 drop Clove oil

5 ml Carrier oil of choice

<u>What To Do</u>

1. Dilute the essential oils in the carrier.

2. Massage the stomach area gently in a clockwise motion.

3. If the pain persists, seek medical advice.

Massage Oil Remedy
2 drops Thyme oil

3 drops Eucalyptus oil

1 drop Pine oil

1 teaspoon Jojoba oil

What To Do

1. Dilute essential oils in Jojoba

2. Massage the back and chest.

Cramp
Cramp is the sudden painful involuntary contraction of a muscle or group of muscles.

3 drops Geranium essential oil

5 ml Evening primrose oil

What To Do

1. Combine oils and massage on the legs.

Bedsores
Bedsores also called pressure sores occur when the body is subjected to constant pressure and irritation. The sores become painful ulcerations and are usually found on the buttocks, elbows and heels of people, especially, bedridden patients.

Bedsore Massage Oil

3 drops Chamomile or Geranium oil

2 drops Tea tree oil

2 drops Lavender oil

4 drops Wheat germ oil

2 drops Frankincense oil

20 ml Evening primrose oil

What To Do

1. Mix all ingredients together.

2. Gently massage the affected area.

3. May be used before bedsore develops.

ORAL HEALTH

Mouth Ulcers

Mouth ulcers are tiny open sores in the mouth, tongue, the roof of the mouth or the mucus membrane inside the cheeks and lips. Ulcers can last from 2 days-3weeks but they heal spontaneously and leave no scar.

<u>What To Do</u>

1. Put 2 drops Tea Tree oil in cotton bud & apply neat dipped to the ulcer.

2. Alternatively, make a mouthwash by adding 2 drops of Tea Tree oil and 5ml salt to 500 ml warm and boiled water.

3. **Power Mouthwash**
    2 drops Thyme oil

    2 drops Geranium oil

    2 drops Peppermint oil

    2 drops Lemon oil

    2 drops Tea tree oil

    1 glass warm water

    10 ml brandy

Combine ingredients& Use as mouthwash. Swish around the mouth and spit.

Gum Strengthener

Firm up gums and prevent gum disease.

1 drop Cinnamon

1 teaspoon of vodka

2 tablespoons of water

<u>What To Do</u>

1. Add the essential oil to vodka and water. Shake the mixture thoroughly.

2. Swish your toothbrush in this mixture. Brush your teeth as usual.

Bad Breath

Bad breath is embarrassing. It could be a symptom of a root problem such as indigestion or improper toxic elimination by the liver or kidney. It could be caused by plaque buildup, decomposing food between the teeth, cigarette smoking and ingestion of strong foods such as garlic and onions.

4 drops Lavender oil

125 ml warm water

5 ml Brandy

<u>What To Do</u>

1. Dilute the oil in the brandy and water and use as mouthwash.

2. Swirl around the mouth after brushing and flossing. Rinse and spit out.

3. Use as needed.

Chapped Lips

Chapped lips can be very painful. It is difficult to keep from licking your sore lips but this process usually increases the pain.

1 drop Chamomile oil

1 drop Neroli oil

2 drops Rose oil

2 drops Geranium oil

20 ml Aloe Vera oil

Mix all the ingredients together in a roller bottle. Apply to lips to ease pain and foster healing.

Toothache

Toothache is usually very painful. It can be regarded as one of the worst pains caused by a minor ailment.

<u>What To Do</u>

1. Put 1 drop of clove essential oil on a cotton bud.

2. Place the cotton bud on the gum around the tooth.

2. Alternatively, place into the crevices on either side.

Massage Oil For Toothache

1 drop Lemon oil

1 drop Clove oil

3 drops Chamomile oil

5 ml vegetable oil

What To Do

1. Dilute in vegetable oil.

2. Massage the cheek and jawbone.

SKIN CARE REMEDIES

For Stretch Marks
3 drops Yarrow

1 teaspoon carrier of choice

Mix and daily rub on the affected areas.

Sunburn Soother
20 drops of lavender oil

1 tablespoon vinegar

200 IU vitamin E oil

4 ounces aloe Vera juice

What To Do

1. Combine all the ingredients. Shake thoroughly before using.

2. store in a spritzer bottle and use as needed.

3. Keep the spray in the refrigerator for extra coolness relief coolness will

Gentle Wart Removal
 Eliminate warts and prevent future outbreaks

1 drop Lemon essential oil (per wart)

Apply undiluted to the affected area directly. Do this several times a day for at 4-5 weeks.

Blemish Blocker

Dab a little of this highly effective mix on your pimple; do not use too often because it may dry out your skin

10 drops Lemon

10 drops Lavender

10 drops Tea Tree

What To Do

1. Combine oils in a dark glass container.

2. Use a cotton swab to apply tiny amounts to skin blemishes.

3. Note: although lemon is not usually applied neat, unlike lavender and tea tree, it is safe for spot-treating" purpose in this preparation.

Easy Facial Toner
5 drops Lavender

5 drops Yarrow

4 oz. Springwater

What To Do

1. Combine all the ingredients. Use as a facial toner.

2. Alternately, add only the essential oils to a simple moisturizer or lotion.

Facial Toner
For oily skin

6 drops juniper berry oil

12 drops lemongrass oil

2 drops ylang ylang oil

1 ounce witch hazel lotion

1 ounce aloe Vera gel

<u>What To Do</u>

1. Combine all the ingredients. Use as a facial toner.

Intensive Blemish Treatment
12 drops tea tree oil

1/2 teaspoon of powdered Oregon grape root, powdered

800 units vitamin E (optional)

A few drops of water

<u>What To Do</u>

1. Add together the herb powder and essential oil, stirring to make a paste.

2. Apply directly as a mask on the blemished area.

3. Allow the paste to dry and remain on your skin for 20- 30 minutes, then rinse off.

4. Repeat again before bedtime, if you wish.

FEVER

A fever is an unusually high body temperature that is often caused by a viral or bacterial infection. Symptoms include shivering, apathy, headache, upward turning of the eyes and dullness. If fevers get too high they could lead to cause seizures or even delirium and this can affect the brain.

Fever Massage Blend

1 drop Rosemary essential oil

2 drops Eucalyptus essential oil

1 drop Tea Tree essential oil

2 drops Peppermint essential oil

2 drops Lavender essential oil

1 drop Black pepper essential oil

15 ml Evening primrose oil

<u>What To Do</u>

1. Add oils together.

2. Massage the top of hands, back of neck, temples and soles of feet.

EYE CARE

Sty

Sty is a temporal swelling on the eyelid. It can develop on the outside as a red sore or itchy spot, which swells and then forms a yellow or pink head. An internal sty is even more painful. The yellowish head is only noticeable when the eyelid is lifted.

1 drop Chamomile essential oil

10 ml rosewater

<u>What To Do</u>

1. Add together and boil.

2. Once cooled, place in a container and shake thoroughly.

3. Strain through a coffee filter and then use the strained mixture to make the compress.

Conjunctivitis Compress

Conjunctivitis is an infection of the conjunctiva. It can be caused by viruses, bacteria, sand, dust or smoke. Symptoms include redness, itching, irritation, burning and tearing.

1 drop of Chamomile oil

5 ml Witch hazel

30 ml Rosewater

<u>What To Do</u>

Combine ingredients and leave for 7-9 hours. Strain through a paper coffee filter. Use as a compress on the closed eyelids.

EAR, NOSE & THROAT

Catarrh

Catarrh is the overproduction and secretion of mucus from the throat and nose. The causes of include colds, flu, bronchitis, hay fever, sinusitis and rhinitis.

1 drop Thyme oil

1 drop Eucalyptus oil

<u>What To Do</u>

1. Drop oils in a bowl of hot water.

2. Drape a towel over your head

3. Inhale for 10 minutes.

Hay Fever

Hay fever is an allergic reaction to pollen or dust. They occur quite spontaneously and usually affect the eyes and the upper respiratory tract. The symptoms include itching eyes, watering eyes, sneezing and runny nose.

<u>What To Do</u>

1. Put 2-3 drops of Tea Tree, Niaouli or Eucalyptus oil on a handkerchief and inhale when an attack occurs.

2. Make a room spray using diluted Eucalyptus oil

Catarrh Rub

3 drops of Tea tree oil

3 drops Rosemary oil

3 drops of Eucalyptus oil

15 ml Evening primrose oil

<u>What To Do</u>

Combine and rub on the chest and the back area.

Pain Relief For Earache

Ear pain is often caused by an infection in the middle-ear. Some of the symptoms are: shooting pains in the ear(s), noises in the ear, fever, a feeling of fullness in the ear, vomiting, nausea and diarrhea.

1 drop Clove oil

5 ml Grape seed oil

<u>What To Do</u>

1. Mix and massage around the ear and neck.

2. If the ear infection was caused by a throat infection, just add 2 drops of Tea tree to a glass of boiled water and then gargle every 2 hours.

Sinusitis Steam Inhalation

Sinusitis is an inflammation of the sinus lining. It could be caused by a flu, cold, tonsillitis, poor mouth hygiene or allergies. The symptoms include nosebleed, nasal congestion, ear pain, fatigue, headache, a mild fever, pain around the eyes or cough.

1 drop Eucalyptus oil

2 drops Peppermint oil

2 drops Rosemary oil

1 drop Thyme oil

Use steam inhalation with these oils.

Massage Oil For Sinusitis

2 drops Eucalyptus oil

3 drops Rosemary oil

2 drops Peppermint oil

1 drop Tea tree oil

3 drops Geranium oil

10 ml carrier oil

<u>What To Do</u>

1. Add essential oils to carrier oil of choice.

2. Massage the nose, around the nose, neck, forehead, cheekbones and in front and behind the ears.

Nosebleed

For a nosebleed without injury or a broken nose, use the remedy below. However, if there is injury or broken nose, see a doctor.

1 drop Lavender oil

3 drops Lemon oil

What To Do

1. Combine oils in a tissue and inhale.

2. Apply an icepack as well.

BODY ACHES & PAINS

Muscle Pain

2 drops Rosemary

2 drops Lavender

4 teaspoons carrier oil of choice

<u>What To Do</u>

1. Combine oils and massage gently onto affected area.

Nerve Pain Oil

Nerves register pain, so when they are damaged, the condition is usually painful. Although injured nerves regenerate slowly, aromatherapy treatments can help to speed up the process.

3 drops marjoram oil

4 drops chamomile oil

2 drops lavender oil

3 drops helichrysum oil (optional)

1 oz vegetable oil

<u>What To Do</u>

1. Combine all ingredients. Apply daily as needed for pain relief.

Back Pain Massage

Back problems can make daily life a misery. Severe pain could be caused by problems with the bone, tendons, ligaments or even a pulled muscle. Other factors that affect the back muscles include, lack of exercise, obesity and incorrect posture. Relieve back pain naturally with this aromatherapy massage:

4 drops cardamom oil

4 drops ginger oil

4 drops wintergreen oil

1 tablespoon sweet oil

What To Do

1. Blend oils and soothingly massage.

Aromatherapy Bath
Soothe tired, aching muscles

8-10 drops essential oils added directly to warm bath water. Soak for 15-20 minutes.

LOWER BLOOD PRESSURE
1 drop Ylang-ylang

2 drops of Clary-Sage

Place these 3 drops on a tissue and inhale.

EMOTIONAL HEALTH

Insomnia Blend

Insomnia means sleeplessness. It is usually caused by anxiety or stress or by physical problems like menopause or pre-menstrual tension. Sleep deprivation may eventually lead to depression chronic agitation, headaches and dizziness. Aromatherapy usually helps.

10 drops lavender oil

15 drops bergamot oil

2 drops ylang ylang oil

10 drops sandalwood oil

3 drops frankincense (optional)

4 ounces vegetable oil

<u>What To Do</u>

1. Combine all ingredients and use combination as massage oil.

2. Put 2 teaspoons in your bath.

3. Alternatively use in a diffuser without the vegetable oil.

Insomnia Remedy

1. Half an hour before bedtime, take a warm bath to which has been added 2-3drops of Lavender or Neroli oil.

2. Alternatively, massage the body with 2-3 drops of Lavender, Clary sage, Ylang ylang or Sandalwood essential oil diluted in carrier oil.

Jetlag

Jetlag occurs when your body's psychological and physiological rhythms are disrupted due to long flights taken. The symptoms include sleep disturbance, fatigue, aching or swollen feet and nausea.

What To Do

1. During the flight, massage your feet with 1 drop of Geranium, Grapefruit or Basil oil diluted with a dash of carrier oil.

2. On arrival, put 10 drops of Lavender oil in your hand and rub on the torso to stay alert and then shower immediately.

3. Revive your mind and body by adding the oils below to a warm bath. Enjoy

2 drops Peppermint essential oil

1 drop Bergamot essential oil

1 drop Rosemary essential oil

1 drop Geranium essential oil

2 drops Neroli essential oil

Release Sexual Energy
2 drop of Sandalwood

2 drops Rosemary

2 drops Jasmine

2 teaspoons jojoba oil

Combine the essential oils in a simmer pot or diffuser.

Comfort the Bereaved
Console the grief-stricken

5 drops Sandalwood

3 drops Rose-Otto

2 teaspoons of jojoba oil

Combine and use as massage

Fatigue Fader
Feel refreshed & renewed

2 drops Lemon

2 drops Peppermint

What To Do

1. In a small bowl, combine essential oils.

2. Dip a cold, moist cloth into the mixture. Lie down; drape cloth across your forehead and temples.

3. Breathe in through your nose and breathe out through your mouth. Do so for 15- 30 minutes.

Concentration Spray

Fight after-lunch sleepiness with this remedy

2 drops Peppermint

3 drops Lemon

3 drops Rosemary

2 cups water

<u>What To Do</u>

1. Add the oils to water and spray around your office or home.

BOOK 4

Essential Oils For Your Pet

47 Safe, Natural And Easy Home Remedies For Fido (Aromatherapy for Dogs)

Coral Miller

INTRODUCTION

Essential Oils And Your Pet

People keep pets for different reasons: for companionship, for protection, for exercise and weight loss or for their looks or specific breed. Whatever valid reason it may be, all pets require effective healthcare and what better, safer, cheaper and all-natural way to go about this than to use essential oils and aromatherapy.

Essential oils are highly concentrated substances extracted from the leaves, bark, bushes, flowers, roots, fruits, shrubs or seeds of plants. They are responsible for providing plants with their powerfully unique scents, while enhancing their immune system and offering the necessary protection. They can be extracted in different ways such as steam distillation, carbon dioxide extraction, solvent extraction or manual expression. Each essential oil comes with its own individual scent, healing benefits, color and chemical properties.

As mentioned earlier, Essential oils are safer, cheaper, and more effective healthcare alternative for fido. Dogs respond very well to it once it is used appropriately. It can be used to treat numerous ailments ranging from allergies and its accompanying symptoms (itchy, dry, flaky skin), skin infections and conditions (wounds, bumps, eczema,), arthritis / muscular issues, respiratory and digestive issues as well as emotional and behavioral concerns (stress, fear, anxiety).

However, for aromatherapy to effectively tackle dog health problems, certain factors must be considered. Topmost on the list is the purity of the essential oils utilized. Only the purest essential oils in the market must be used. The essentials oils must have a "Therapeutic Grade" rating. If you use aromatherapy grade or perfume quality oils for topical application, for example, you may be doing more harm than good because the oils are distilled using solvents. Pure therapeutic grade oils are steam distilled and do not contain any chemicals.

The price indicates its level of purity. Pure therapeutic essential oils are usually more costly. So if you see cheaper essential oils in the market, do not buy as they may be adulterated. The oils must also be bottled in cobalt, violet or amber glass bottles.

Another important factor is dilution and dosage. Dilution has to do with the amount of essential oils that is present in a blend while dosage is the amount of the blend that is administered to the dog such as drops.

Diluting Essential Oils For Dogs

Essential oils must be diluted according to the size of the dog. For small dogs that are between 5-15 pounds, essential oil dilution ratio is 90%. For small-medium dogs that are between 16-30 pounds, the dilution ratio is 75%. Medium dogs, 31-50 pounds would have a 50% dilution of the essential oil.

s/n	Size of Dog	Weight (lb)	Essential Oil Dilution Ratio
1	small dogs	5- 15 lb	90%
2	small- medium dogs	16-30 lb	75%
3	medium dogs	31-50 lb	50%
4	large dogs	51-89 lb	25%
5	extra large dogs	90lb and over	undiluted

The amount of dilution also depends on the type of essential oil. Lavender and roman chamomile oils for instance are gentle and so may not require much dilution. Lavender can even be used without dilution. Strong essential oils like oregano, clove and thyme must always be diluted accordingly.

The response should also be monitored. Response either positive or negative occurs immediately or several days later. If there is no response, try another essential oil. If there is a negative response such as mild pinkness of the skin or mild watering of the eyes, let your pet rest for 24-48 hours then try another essential oil.

This is another reason you should use 100% pure essential oils, it is safe for dogs and usually do not cause adverse effects. If using oil for the first time, introduce it to the dog in small amounts to see if it upsets him. He shows this by panting, drooling or whining. Start with gentle oil and then and work up to the stronger ones.

Always dilute with a pure carrier and not water. Also, correct adverse reaction with pure carrier oil by using to wash the affected area. For dosage, small dogs require fewer amounts of diluted oils while bigger dogs will need a larger amount.

Essential Oils Benefits for Fido

1. It is non-toxic to the body. It is safe to apply and leave no side effects.

2. It is easy to use. Dogs can inhale essential oils directly from the bottle or from your hand. You can also apply directly on their paw or body.

3. Extremely versatile, essential oils address a wide range of issues such as motion sickness, tick removal and stomach problems. They are very effective as well.

4. They increase alertness for pets as they age. They help to reestablish old habits so the pets maintain their level of alertness even as they grow old. Cedarwood, frankincense, sandalwood, lavender, vetiver and lemon oils are examples.

5. They are great training aids for emotions. They can be used to calm anxiety and to make dogs concentrate.

6. They improve coat and skin. Essential oils help the skin to regenerate, its antioxidant effects helps to restore health to the coat.

7. They are safe cleaning agents. There is no fear of your pets ingesting caustic cleaners while drinking from toilet bowls or licking areas where such cleaners are used. Lemon, rosemary, and eucalyptus oils are examples.

8. Helps to eliminates odors. Use essential oils to eliminate pet odors and stains and keep your home smelling nice all day long.

Safe Essential Oils For Dogs

While essential oils provide a range of treatments for your pets, they are not all safe for your dogs. Below are a few popular oils that you can safely use on your dogs.

Lavender

A "must-have" for your dog, lavender oil is a good first aid that is extremely safe and gentle. It is antibacterial and helps to treat common animal ailments such as skin irritations and itches. It calms and soothes. It can be used diluted or undiluted.

Bergamot

Antifungal and soothing, this essential oil helps to fight ear infections caused by bacterial overgrowth or yeast. However, it can cause photosensitization so your pet must stay away from the sun after use.

Chamomile, Roman

It is analgesic and antispasmodic. It helps to soothe the central nervous system. It provides relief from cramps, muscle pains and teething pain. It is very important for dogs.

Helichrysum

Anti-inflammatory and analgesic oil, helichrysum is an excellent skin regenerator. It is great for skin conditions such as eczema. It reduces bleeding in accidents. It helps heal scars and bruises and it is effective for pain relief.

Niaouli

Although Niaouli has powerful antibacterial properties, it is gentle on the skin. It works wonderfully on ear infections and skin troubles caused by allergies.

Peppermint

Antispasmodic, peppermint stimulates circulation. It can be combined with ginger essential oil to effectively treat motion sickness. It also helps with arthritis, sprains and strains. Repel insects as well.

Geranium

Antifungal, it is gentle and safe, good fungal ear infections and skin irritations. It is an effective tick repellant.

Valerian

It helps to calm nerves and thus good for treating anxiety in dogs.

Eucalyptus Radiata

It is antiviral and anti-inflammatory. An effective expectorant, it provides relief from chest congestion. It also repels fleas.

German Chamomile

This oil works well on burns, stings and good for allergic reactions.

Essential Oil Precautions With Dogs

- Always dilute essential oils with a carrier oil like olive oil or coconut oil. To guide you, add about 10 to15 drops of essential oils to 15 ml (1/2 oz) of carrier oil.

- Use cautiously with pregnant dogs, puppies under 10 weeks of age or very old dogs. As a matter of fact, check with your vet before using on pregnant dogs.

- Avoid nose, eyes, anal, anal area and genital areas.

- Always use 100% therapeutic grade essential oils that is pure and non- adulterated.

- Do not use oils on seizure-prone or epileptic dogs.

- Do not try to treat seriously injured dogs. Consult your vet.

- Less is More! Being conservative with essential oil is safer than being liberal. Dogs' olfactory sensitivity is reported to be about 100 times greater than humans. They can detect odorant molecules at a really lower concentration.

- Do not use these oils on dogs: pennyroyal, wormwood, rue, horseradish, birch, wintergreen, camphor, clove leaf, cassia and anise.

- Always wash your hands after applying oils so it doesn't accidentally get into your eyes.

- Do not add your 100% pure essential oils to synthetic shampoos, laundry soaps, detergents. Use all natural bases instead.

How To Apply Essential Oils To Dogs

Topically

Topical application is the most common of all as it provides the greatest benefits. The oils are applied directly to the area (s) of concern and are quickly absorbed into the bloodstream. The ears, toes, pads and spine of dogs are common examples. Essential oils can also be applied directly to the wound or via massage. However, avoid getting it into the eyes, nose, anal and genital areas. The oils can be added to shampoos, ointments, conditioners, salves, etc as well.

Aromatically

Essential oils can be applied aromatically via inhalation and diffusion. You can put a drop of essential oil on his collar or on the dog bed. He can even inhale from your hands. Spritzers or sprays can also be used by mixing essential oil and water and spraying on fur.

A diffuser helps to evaporate the oils which are then inhaled by the dog. For your pet to inhale and absorb the essential oils very well, leave the diffuser on for at least 30 minutes. You may do this procedure twice daily for a week so as to get positive result.

Internally

Never administer essential oils to your pets internally unless under supervision of a veterinarian. Remember they are highly concentrated and potent so take extreme care so you do not administer overdose. Even when you get a vet's approval, do not administer more than 1 drop in an empty capsule for your dog. The oils must also be Certified Pure Therapeutic Grade.

ESSENTIAL OIL DOG BATH RECIPES

Calming Shampoo
Make your dog relax after a bath

What You Need

2 drops Vetiver essential oil

4 drops Petitgrain essential oil

3 drops valerian essential oil

2 drops sweet orange essential oil

3 drops sweet marjoram essential oil

8 oz (240ml) all natural shampoo base

Directions

1. Add oils to shampoo.

2. Shake thoroughly and use.

Puppy Shampoo
What You Need

5 drops geranium essential oil

5 drops petitgrain essential oil

2 drops rose essential oil

2 drops ylang ylang essential oil

2 drops roman chamomile essential oil

8 oz (240ml) all natural shampoo base

Directions

1. Add oils to shampoo.

2. Shake thoroughly and use.

Tick Repelling Shampoo
What You Need

2 drops rosewood essential oil

3 drops lavender essential oil

2 drops geranium essential oil

2 drops myrrh essential oil

1 drops bay leaf essential oil

2 drops opoponax essential oil

8 oz (240ml) all natural shampoo base

Directions

1. Add oils to shampoo.

2. Shake thoroughly and use.

Flea/ Insect Repelling Shampoo
What You Need

2 drops citronella essential oil

4 drops clary sage essential oil

4 drops lemon essential oil

8 drops peppermint essential oil

8 oz (240ml) all natural shampoo base

Directions

1. Add oils to shampoo.

2. Shake thoroughly and use.

Spicy Deodorant Shampoo
What You Need

4 drops atlas cedarwood essential oil

2 drops patchouli essential oil

4 drops rosemary essential oil

3 drops vetiver essential oil

8 oz (240ml) all natural shampoo base

Directions

1. Add oils to shampoo.

2. Shake thoroughly and use.

Tender Floral
What You Need

6 drops petitgrain essential oil

4 drops lavender essential oil

4 drops rose essential oil

2 drops ylang ylang, essential oil

8 oz (240ml) all natural shampoo base

Directions

1. Add oils to shampoo.

2. Shake thoroughly and use.

Citrus Refreshing Shampoo
3 drops grapefruit essential oil

3 drops lemon essential oil

3 drops Lime essential oil

3 drops Sweet Orange essential oil

3 drops mandarin essential oil

8 oz (240ml) all natural shampoo base

Directions

1. Add oils to shampoo.

2. Shake thoroughly and use.

Herbal Fresh Shampoo
What You Need

4 drops clary sage essential oil

4 drops sweet basil essential oil

4 drops coriander seed essential oil

4 drops lavender essential oil

8 oz (240ml) all natural shampoo base

Directions

1. Add oils to shampoo.

2. Shake thoroughly and use.

ESSENTIAL OILS FOR DOGS' EARS

Lavender Wax Cleanser

You need to clean dog ears regularly, at least once in a month. This is because Dog ear wax can lead to other ear problems. Besides, it smells terrible and if your dog is outside all day, the dirt can accumulate quickly.

What You Need

5 drops lavender

1 tsp pure witch hazel or vegetable oil

Directions

1. Combine ingredients in a dark bottle.

2. Place several drops on a cotton swab.

3. Remove the surface dirt and then gently remove the wax.

4. Do not stick swab down the ear canal.

5. The mixture can be used for 2-3 cleanings

Wax In The Ear Canal

What do you do when the wax accumulates is the ear canal?

1. Apply 4 drops of the oil mixture above into the ear canal

2. Massage the exterior area of the ear.

3. Your dog will start to shake vigorously but do not worry about this as it will help to bring up the ear wax to the surface where it can easily be cleaned out.

4. Hold your nose! The wax will smell really bad. With regular cleaning however, there will be no need to do this often.

Doggie Ear Mites
What You Need

1 drop purifying essential oil

1 drop peppermint essential oil

Cotton ball

Directions

1. Apply oils to cotton ball

2. Swab just the inner ear.

Dog Ear Infection
What You Need

5 drops Melaleuca

5 drops Lavender

5 drops Geranium

1 tbsp coconut oil

Directions

1. Combine all ingredients

2. Clean the ear with a natural cleaner and then use a Q-tip to carefully rub mixture in the ear.

3. Do this two times daily until the infection clears up.

Power Ear Infection Blend
For dogs with long ears

What You Need

4 drops lavender essential oil

7 drops bergamot essential oil

3 drops roman chamomile essential oil

2 drops niaouli or tea tree essential oil

1/2 oz. (15 ml) carrier oil

Directions

1. Combine oils in a dark glass bottle.

2. Drop 2-3 drops into dog's ear canal with a dropper. Massage outside of the ear gently and then use a cotton ball to clean the ear.

3. The dirt in the ear should loosen and wash out. This reduces the risk of ear infections.

SKIN AND COAT ISSUES

Dog Burns
What You Need

3-5 drops Lavender Essential Oil

Directions

1. Make a cold water compress to cool the burn.

2. Apply the oil as soon as possible.

Deodorizing Spray
Use on your dogs if he stinks from prolong outside play. The result is a wonderful smell that will stay with him for days.

What You Need

5 drops Lavender Essential Oil

15 drops Purification Essential Oil

Pinch of Salt

5 oz Water

Directions

1. Add the essential oils to the salt, stirring gently. Now add the water.

2. Spray your dog lightly.

3. This recipe is for dogs weighing over 60 pounds. For smaller dogs, double the amount water for a larger dilution ratio.

Dog Abscess

What You Need

2 drops Melaleuca essential oil

2 drops Lavender essential oil

Directions

1. Clean the wound area.

2. Apply Melaleuca essential oil directly on the abscess. Apply several times in a day.

3. Once pus is gone, apply the lavender oil to speed up healing.

Calming Mist Spray

Use this recipe to freshen up your dog's coat and remove odors after a long playing day outside.

What You Need

5-10 drops lavender

5-10 drops roman chamomile

10 oz water

Directions

1. Combine in a glass spray bottle.

2. Shake well before application.

Rich Fragrant Shampoo
For dry skin & fleas

What You Need

3 drops peppermint essential oil

2 drops roman chamomile

3 drops lavender essential oil

2 drops Purification

1 drops cedar wood

1 tablespoons castile soap

¼ tsp vitamin E

1 cup water

2 drops citronella (optional, for fleas)

Directions

1. Combine all ingredients in a glass jar. Mixture will be watery with little suds.

2. However, it is gentle and works perfectly. Your dog will smell great for days!

3. To make this a flea and tick shampoo, just add 2drops of citronella essential oil to it.

4. This recipe is for dogs weighing over 60 pounds. For smaller dogs, double the amount of water for a larger dilution ratio.

Wound Blend
For minor cuts, bruises, scrapes and insect bites

What You Need

1 drop Helichrysum

4 drops Lavender

2 drops Niaouli

3 drops sweet marjoram

1/2 oz. (15 ml) olive oil or jojoba oil

Directions

1. Combine and store in a dark glass bottle.

2. Use as needed.

Dog Growths
1. Apply 1 drop Frankincense directly on the growth.

2. Apply undiluted 2 times daily.

Doggie Anti-Itch Blend
To alleviate itching and reduce redness.

What You Need

5 drops Lavender essential oil

5 drops Roman Chamomile

2-3 drops Frankincense (optional)

5 oz olive or jojoba oil

3 drops of vitamin E

Directions

1. Combine in a glass dropper bottle.

2. To help soothe the skin, apply 2- to 4 drops to the spot two times daily. For itching apply as needed.

3. This recipe is for dogs weighing over 60 pounds. For smaller dogs, double the amount of carrier oils in the recipe.

Insect Bite Blend
What You Need

10 drops lavender essential oil

2 drops thyme essential oil

4 drops eucalyptus radiata

3 drops German chamomile essential oil

20 drops V-6 vegetable oil complex

Directions:

1. Combine all ingredients in dark glass bottle, turning gently to mix.

2. Apply 1 or 2 drops 2 to 4 times a day for relief.

3. This recipe has only been tested on dogs between 35-55 pounds. Adjust recipe for dogs below 20 pounds or above 60 pounds.

Itchy Skin Remedy
What You Need

7 drops lavender essential oil

2 drops German chamomile essential oil

3 drops geranium essential oil

3 drops carrot seed

Directions:

1. Combine oils and add to 8 oz. (240 ml) of an all-natural shampoo

2. Alternatively add blend to or to 1/2 oz. of any carrier oil.

3. Apply topically on dog's affected skin areas.

Bad Odor Remedy
Keep your dog smelling fresh and lovely all day long!

What You Need

2 drops Chamomile Roman essential oil

2 drops Geranium essential oil

7-8 drops Lavender essential oil

3 drops Sweet Marjoram essential oil

8 oz. (240 ml) all-natural shampoo

Directions:

Combine oils in the shampoo

Power Odor Spray
This quick-and-easy spray will get rid of that nasty dog smell fast!

10 drops lavender essential oil

3 drops eucalyptus essential oil

6 drops peppermint essential oil

6 drops sweet orange essential oil

1 cup distilled water

Directions:

1. Add oils to water

2. Mix thoroughly in a spray bottle.

FLEAS AND TICKS

Natural Tick Spritzer
What You Need

1 cup distilled water

2 drops palo santo essential oil

4 drops grapefruit essential oil

2 drops geranium essential oil

1 drop myrrh essential oil

1 drop peppermint essential oil

1 drop castile soap (emollient)

Directions

1. Combine all in a spray bottle, shaking well. Spritz as needed.

2. It is suitable for horses too.

Oregano Tick Removal

1. Apply 1drop of oregano essential oil directly on the tick.

2. The tick should release its grip.

3. If the area is unreachable, place the oil on a cotton swab and then swab the tick.

Flea Control
What You Need

3 drops lemongrass essential oil

3 drops lavender essential oil

3 drops eucalyptus globulus

3 drops lemon essential oil

4 ounces distilled water

4-ounce dark glass spray bottle

Directions

1. Combine all ingredients in a spray bottle, shaking well.

2. Spray on dogs between 35-55 pounds. Adjust recipe for dogs under 20 or over 60 pounds.

3. Rub on areas in the home where fleas usually congregate.

Tick Repellent

3 drops bay Leaf essential oil

5 drops geranium essential oil

7 drops lavender essential oil

1/2 oz. (15 ml) sweet almond oil

Directions

Combine and apply 2-3 drops to the tail, neck, chest, back, and legs of your dog.

Flea and Deodorizing Collar
Instant flea and allergy collar!

What You Need

2 drops lavender essential oil

2 drops citronella essential oil

2 drops peppermint essential oil

2 drops purification essential oil

⅓ cup purified water

Directions

1. Combine all in a small bowl and soak dog's collar in it.

2. Try not to submerge any plastic pieces as essential oils can degrade plastic.

3. Leave collar to dry and then put it on dog!

4. Store the remaining liquid in a mason jar for use every two weeks.

5. This recipe is for dogs weighing over 60 pounds. For smaller dogs, double the amount of water in the recipe for a larger dilution ratio.

Anti Fleas Shampoo
What You Need

Any doggy all- natural shampoo of choice

1-2 drops of lemongrass essential oil

Directions

1. Add the oil to the shampoo and use on pet.

2. You can also add a few drops of the oil to your dog's beddings and blankets when washing or rinsing.

Mosquito Repellent

Mosquitoes transmit heartworm disease in dogs so protect your dogs from them with this homemade repellent.

What You Need

10 drops Myrrh essential oil

20 drops Citronella essential oil

10 drops Rose Geranium essential oil

10 drops Lemongrass essential oil

8 ounces Aloe Vera juice

Directions

1. Combine all in a sprintzer and sprintz on dog's coat daily.

2. Be careful to avoid the eye area.

ESSENTIAL OILS FOR EMOTIONS

Like humans, dogs have emotions which are very real to them. Use essential oils to address such emotions like dog anxiety, separation anxiety, fear and stress. They can also be used to calm dogs during thunderstorms and to enliven them during times of loss, depression or separation.

For Calming Dogs
What You Need

1 drop Lavender or Roman Chamomile essential oil

1 drop carrier oil

Directions

1. Mix and rub on dog pads, ears whenever you perceive your dog is stressed.

2. You can also comb through fur.

For Girl Crazy Dogs
Help your dog stay calm and focus with this recipe.

2-3 drops marjoram essential oil

Rub gently on fur

For Hyperactive Dogs
What You Need

2 drops roman Chamomile essential oil

5 drops lavender essential oil

2 drops bergamot essential oil

3 drops Sweet Marjoram essential oil

3 drops Valerian essential oil

1/2 oz. (15 ml) almond oil or olive oil

Directions

1. Combine all ingredients and then rub 2 to 3 drops between your hands.

2. Apply to dog's inner thighs, the edge of his ears or between the toes.

Anxiety Oil Blend
To calm dogs who are afraid of new places, people or things as well as those who suffer from separation anxiety (when an otherwise gentle dog becomes overwrought and destructive when you are not at home) and noise anxiety.

What You Need

2 drops clary sage essential oil

3 drops sweet marjoram essential oil

5 drops lavender essential oil

3 drops valerian essential oil

1/2 oz. (15 ml) jojoba oil, olive oil or sweet almond oil

Directions

1. Combine all ingredients and then rub 2 to 3 drops between your hands.

2. Apply to dog's inner thighs, the edge of his ears or between the toes.

For Nervous Exhaustion
Rub 2 to 3 drops lavender essential oil on dog's tummy

Calming Powder Blend
For stressed dogs and those with anxiety issues

What You Need

3 parts lavender essential oil

2 parts Melissa essential oil

2 parts bergamot essential oil

1 part ylang ylang essential oil

Baking soda, cornstarch or rice flour

Directions

1. Combine the essential oils. Use 12 to 15 drops of the blend per cup of baking soda.

2. Alternatively, mix baking soda and rice flour together and use per cup for 12 to 15 drops essential oil blend flour.

3. Shake or stir to mix well.

How To Use

If your dog is stressed during a car ride, sprinkle the lavender powder blend on a blanket and put it in the cage with the dog.

If your dog suffers from separation anxiety when you are away, sprinkle the powder on any of your old clothes and place it on your dog's bed. Your old clothes emit your smell which reassures your dog while the calming effects of the oil powder blend helps him relax.

ESSENTIAL OIL FOR BONE ISSUES

Joint Pain Relief Blend

1 drop oregano essential oil

5 drops peppermint essential oil

10 drops helichrysum essential oil

30 drops Idaho balsam fir essential oil

Directions

1. Combine all ingredients in dark glass bottle, shaking gently to mix.

2. Apply 2 to 3 drops to the affected joint thrice daily for relief.

3. This recipe has only been tested on dogs between 35-55 pounds. Adjust recipes for dogs below 20 pounds or above 60 pounds.

Doggie Aging Ointment
As dogs get older, they suffer from aches and pains. This recipe will be helpful for them.

What You Need

3 tbsp coconut oil

3 drops peppermint essential oil

2 drops balsam fir essential oil

3 drops lavender essential oil

2 drops copaiba essential oil

Directions

Make into an ointment and then rub onto the pad of the foot to absorb quickly into the blood stream.

Arthritis Relief

What You Need

3 drops Valerian essential oil

6 drops Helichrysum essential oil

2 drops Ginger essential oil

4 drops Peppermint essential oil

1/2 oz. (15 ml) olive oil, jojoba oil or sweet almond oil

Directions

1. Combine all and massage on dog's sore joints.

2. Apply 1-2 drops on his inner ear tips too.

ESSENTIAL OILS FOR MICELLANEOUS ISSUES

Immune Support for Allergens
What You Need

1 drop lavender

1 drop peppermint

1 drop lemon

Directions

1. Combine ingredients in an empty capsule.

2. Put it in dog's food or give him directly to swallow.

3. Consult with your vet before use.

Sunburned Nosed Dog
What You Need

1-2 drops lavender essential oil

1tsp carrier oil

Directions

Combine and dab on nose for relief.

Sinus Infections
Use this blend to relieve your dog of nasal congestion caused by sinus infection.

What You Need

1/2 oz. (15 ml) jojoba oil

5 drops eucalyptus essential oil

5 drops Myrrh essential oil

5 drops Ravensare essential oil

Directions

Combine in a dark glass bottle.

To Use

- Massage 5-7 drops onto dog's chest and neck or place on a cloth bandanna.
- Alternatively, add several drops of it to the dog's bedding or…
- Let the dog lay on the bathroom floor when you are about to shower. Drop 6-10 drops of the blend onto the shower floor. The steam and vaporized oil will work together to clear the dog's sinus congestion.
- Alternatively, add the only essential oils and not the carrier oils to a diffuser and diffuse for 5 minutes at a time, several times a day.

Carsick Dogs/ Colic
Rub 2-3 drops peppermint EO on the tummy.

For Brain Health Support
What You Need

1 drop Frankincense

1 drop lavender

Directions

Apply the Frankincense on spine and the lavender on paws.

Respiratory Support
<u>What You Need</u>

1 drop lime

1 drop thyme

<u>Directions</u>

Combine and apply to the paws.

Dog With A High Fever
<u>What You Need</u>

2-4 drops peppermint essential oil

1 tsp carrier oil

<u>Directions</u>

1. Combine and sprinkle on dog's body.

2. Wrap cool towel over him

Motion Sickness
<u>What You Need</u>

6 drops ginger essential oil

6 to 8 drops peppermint essential oil

1/2 oz. (15 ml) olive oil or jojoba oil

<u>Directions</u>

1. Combine and apply onto dog's belly and the inside tip of ears.

2. Also, add 2 to 3 drops to a cotton ball and place in front of the air vent in the car. Scent will then circulate in the car.

Made in the USA
Monee, IL
17 January 2020